Helen Beare was born in 19...

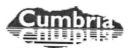

...artered

...ice established by him in 1989, until
1996 when Neil's cancer was diagnosed. She has written
two other books for Sheldon Press, *How to Avoid
Business Failure* (1993) and *Your Own Business: From
Concept to Success* (1995).

Neil Priddy was born in Essex in 1960. He lived in both
the UK and Brussels before taking a degree in politics,
philosophy and economics at Oxford University. In 1985
he qualified as a chartered accountant and worked for
both small and large firms of accountants in London
before establishing his own practice near Buckingham in
1989. The business was sold in 1996 when Neil was
diagnosed with testicular cancer. After an eighteen-
month battle against his disease, Neil died in December
1997, shortly before the completion of this book.

Overcoming Common Problems Series

For a full list of titles please contact
Sheldon Press, Marylebone Road, London NW1 4DU

The Assertiveness Workbook
A plan for busy women
JOANNA GUTMANN

Birth Over Thirty Five
SHEILA KITZINGER

Body Language
How to read others' thoughts by their
gestures
ALLAN PEASE

Body Language in Relationships
DAVID COHEN

Cancer – A Family Affair
NEVILLE SHONE

Coping Successfully with Hayfever
DR ROBERT YOUNGSON

Coping Successfully with Migraine
SUE DYSON

Coping Successfully with Pain
NEVILLE SHONE

**Coping Successfully with Your Irritable
Bowel**
ROSEMARY NICOL

Coping with Anxiety and Depression
SHIRLEY TRICKETT

Coping with Breast Cancer
DR EADIE HEYDERMAN

Coping with Bronchitis and Emphysema
DR TOM SMITH

Coping with Chronic Fatigue
TRUDIE CHALDER

Coping with Depression and Elation
DR PATRICK McKEON

Curing Arthritis Diet Book
MARGARET HILLS

Curing Arthritis – The Drug-Free Way
MARGARET HILLS

Depression
DR PAUL HAUCK

Divorce and Separation
Every woman's guide to a new life
ANGELA WILLANS

**Everything Parents Should Know About
Drugs**
SARAH LAWSON

Good Stress Guide, The
MARY HARTLEY

Heart Attacks – Prevent and Survive
DR TOM SMITH

Helping Children Cope with Grief
ROSEMARY WELLS

How to Improve Your Confidence
DR KENNETH HAMBLY

How to Interview and Be Interviewed
MICHELE BROWN AND GYLES
BRANDRETH

How to Keep Your Cholesterol in Check
DR ROBERT POVEY

How to Pass Your Driving Test
DONALD RIDLAND

**How to Start a Conversation and Make
Friends**
DON GABOR

How to Write a Successful CV
JOANNA GUTMANN

Hysterectomy
SUZIE HAYMAN

The Irritable Bowel Diet Book
ROSEMARY NICOL

Overcoming Guilt
DR WINDY DRYDEN

The Parkinson's Disease Handbook
DR RICHARD GODWIN-AUSTEN

Talking About Anorexia
How to cope with life without starving
MAROUSHKA MONRO

Think Your Way to Happiness
DR WINDY DRYDEN AND JACK
GORDON

Overcoming Common Problems

The Cancer Guide for Men

Helen Beare and Neil Priddy

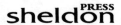

First published in Great Britain in 1999 by
Sheldon Press, SPCK, Marylebone Road, London NW1 4DU

© Helen Beare and Neil Priddy 1999

British Library Cataloguing-in-Publication Data
A catalogue for this book is available from the British Library

ISBN 0–85969–793–2

Photoset by Deltatype Limited, Birkenhead, Merseyside
Printed in Great Britain by
Biddles Ltd, Guildford and King's Lynn

Contents

Foreword

It is an honour to write the foreword for this book. Neil Priddy and his wife Helen are to be congratulated on writing an excellent account of their experience with cancer, from both a personal and a patient's point of view. I first met Neil after he was diagnosed with cancer and was struck, despite the circumstances, by his positive and cheerful personality. I was impressed from the outset by Neil and Helen's practical approach, optimism and realism about the illness. All members of the medical team came to know Neil well and were particularly fond of him. Unfortunately, though he was initially successful in getting rid of the cancer, it quickly returned. This time intensive efforts to eradicate the cancer, which Neil together with Helen faced with great courage, were unsuccessful. As a doctor, even though one has to maintain equanimity, I felt very sad that in Neil's case we had failed to cure him.

It was during one of his stays in hospital that I learned that he and Helen were planning to write about their experience. Neil felt strongly that, because there was a shortage of books on cancers specific to men, it was necessary to raise the profile of these diseases. This is important as one such disease, testicular cancer, occurs at a young age and with appropriate treatment is curable. Prostate cancer also occurs only in men and is rapidly becoming a health priority as men live longer. Although excellent information is available through organizations such as BACUP in the UK, a personal account such as Neil's has immediate resonance for another man with a similar disease. This book, which was started during Neil's treatment, has been completed by Helen with great fortitude.

As a doctor, I found the book illuminating in several ways. It is clear that sometimes patients' concerns are simply not picked up by the medical team and the system. These instances have been illustrated elegantly and – to Neil's and Helen's credit – charitably, without rancour. I was impressed by the lucid style in which terminology and jargon often used by medical teams are explained. For example, the book distinguishes between the types of cancers where the intent of treatment is to cure and others where it is palliative. Learning how to cope with all aspects of life after a diagnosis of cancer is seldom easy.

The book outlines key stages in a patient's journey with cancer – the numbness that follows diagnosis, fluctuating emotions through treatment and, in this instance, the acceptance of the reality of death. Helen's and Neil's personal observations during Neil's illness are poignant but instructive. They emphasize the importance of obtaining information about cancer in order to cope with it adequately. These chapters describing their own experience contain helpful advice for other patients on many aspects of life – such as relationships and daily living, work and finances – which often undergo great change after a cancer diagnosis.

I am sure that Neil would have been proud of *The Cancer Guide for Men*. It is a testament to his belief that 'where there's a will, there's a way'. This book is an important legacy that I believe will benefit many other patients with cancer.

Dr T. S. Ganesan MD, PhD MNAMS, FRCP
Consultant Medical Oncologist
The Churchill Hospital, Oxford

Introduction

Our motivation for writing this book was Neil's diagnosis of testicular cancer in June 1996. We were offered scant verbal information or help in finding either medical or general literature about his cancer, treatment or coping and living with the disease. After the shock of diagnosis, we began almost immediately to search out information for ourselves. We found leaflets and pamphlets and one or two autobiographical works, but it became clear to us that while much has been written about cancer from a female perspective, there were no books which dealt specifically with men and cancer. In one medical bookshop we were cheerfully informed, 'No, you won't find anything like that because it's not women's issues, is it?' So we decided to do it ourselves.

This book is about coping and living with cancer: how it affects your daily life, your relationships – every aspect of your life, in fact – and how you can confront these issues. There are no rules for coping with cancer. What we have done is to look at some of the ways in which coping can be made easier, both practically and emotionally. We did not set out to provide detailed information about particular cancers or treatments because good, basic factual literature does exist. We have included some description of the cancers which commonly affect men and their treatments but we wanted to put this in a broader context.

The early chapters provide descriptions of how cancer develops, of the cancers which commonly affect men and of the conventional forms of treatment. The remainder of the book looks at coping as effectively as possible with cancer from a number of different angles: dealing with your medical team; getting through the early stages after diagnosis; the effects of living with cancer on your personal relationships and daily life; financial and other practical issues.

As non-medics, we are indebted to Dr T. S. Ganesan of the ICRF Medical Oncology Unit at the Churchill Hospital in Oxford and Dr J. Chester of St James' Hospital in Leeds for checking the factual accuracy of the medical information in the book.

We hope that if you or someone close to you has recently been diagnosed with cancer, you will find a useful factual background in the first three chapters and equally important information about ways of coping in the rest of the book. If you already have some experience of living with cancer, the 'coping' sections of the book may feel more familiar, but we hope that you will find fresh ideas to renew your strength and resolve.

Neil fought his cancer with great energy and determination because he was that kind of man. It is not the only way, and it is important for all men to find ways which suit them best. Neil's treatment was at first apparently very successful, but he suffered a relapse in early 1997 and after a long year of continuing treatment, he died in December 1997. He felt he was hugely unlucky: relatively old for this type of cancer (he was 35 when diagnosed with a testicular teratoma) and desperately unfortunate to be in the small proportion of men for whom treatment is not effective. This was his way of rationalizing his disease. You may feel differently about your own cancer.

This book was almost complete when Neil died, and stands as a testament to his deep conviction that the most appalling situations can be made easier to live with if we are willing to confront them, talk about them and take what control we can over them. He also hoped that others would benefit both from our personal experience and from our contact with other men living with cancer.

While this book was born out of a tremendous personal motivation, we received invaluable and enthusiastic support from a variety of sources. There are many individuals – family, friends, patients and medical staff alike – who contributed to our views on coping with cancer by sharing with us their own perceptions and experiences. We would particularly like to thank Dr T. S. Ganesan for his support, for writing the foreword, for checking the book from a medical standpoint and for his suggestions and comments from a doctor's point of view. Thanks are also due to Dr John Chester for checking the text for medical accuracy at an early stage and for his feedback. We are especially grateful to Judith Beare who read and commented on the book and offered suggestions based on her close involvement in our experience. Finally, we owe much to Neil's parents, Jan and Derek Priddy, for all their love, support and encouragement.

Helen Beare

1
Male health

Hearing the word 'cancer' used by a doctor for the first time is a moment no patient ever forgets. The very nature of cancer makes it particularly difficult to face, let alone to discuss rationally in the early stages when fear and shock may be your only recognizable emotions.

Most of us take good health and fitness for granted and assume that our bodies will function happily with little or no special attention well into advanced years. With constant medical advances and new, effective treatments for a whole range of conditions, we also tend to expect that any health problems we do encounter will be quickly resolved. As a result, we simply don't anticipate that ill-health will have any major or long-term impact on our lives. It would be foolish to spend our lives in a constant state of fear about our health, but our expectations are now so high that when serious ill-health does strike, we are rarely prepared to cope with it.

Attitudes to ill-health

In our society, we are constantly faced with images which teach us that we should strive for peak physical fitness. We learn that good physical health is highly desirable, not just from the point of view of our personal well-being, but also because of the overall picture it promotes of us as individuals: strength and good health are prized and admired.

At the same time, women's health issues have been receiving increasing attention in newspapers and magazines, in books and on television and radio programmes.

Women have been positively encouraged to learn more about, and to take responsibility for, their overall physical well-being. This doesn't just mean keeping fit through physical exercise and by eating a balanced diet, but encourages self-awareness and attendance at screening programmes, for example. Furthermore, responsibility for health matters within the family has tended to remain the province of women. Men, in general, are not as comfortable talking about health issues, whether minor or serious, as many women. This is not a matter for criticism so much as a reflection of the way in which attitudes towards health in our society have evolved.

And there is some evidence of changing attitudes. Until relatively recently, the specific health needs of men have been somewhat neglected. Now there are numerous general interest health/fitness magazines for men.

Although their health and medical issues are often covered from a general 'lifestyle' viewpoint ('look after your body and become more attractive'), specifically male medical matters such as prostate problems and testicular self-examination do receive an airing alongside the broader issues. These magazines are largely aimed at and read by the younger adult male population, leaving a gap in older age-ranges which is less easily filled.

A serious hurdle for many men to overcome is the traditional social pressure to be 'strong' where physical (not to mention emotional) health is concerned. This perceived need to be – and to be *seen* to be – strong is a major obstacle to an open and constructive approach to health problems. Many of us know of men who lead largely sedentary lives yet take enormous pride in over-exerting themselves in the gym or on the squash court, followed by large quantities of beer in the bar afterwards. These men seem to have a need to proclaim to their peers that regardless of their general fitness, their bodies can withstand the same exertions as when they were 18 years old. External pressures to be seen to be strong can manifest themselves in many different ways, from a denial of illness to an obsession with physical fitness regimes.

The same underlying problem is evident in many men's reluctance to seek help if they become unwell. A certain pride in never visiting the doctor, or declaring that 'I've never had a day off work sick in 30 years' is fine – up to a point. It is still very important to recognize when a visit to the doctor is called for, or when a few days off work would lead to a faster recovery from a niggling virus. There is still a tendency for an admission of illness to be equated with unacceptable and 'unmanly' weakness. Many men would rather suffer in silence than admit to ill-health and run the risk, however unconsciously, of being perceived as weak. Sometimes, different attitudes can prevail depending upon the nature of the problem. An injury sustained while involved in a very physical activity – a dislocated shoulder on the rugby field, for example – is regarded somehow more positively than a bad bout of 'flu. The former is still connected with a display of physical strength, the latter with physical weakness.

For similar reasons, even admitting to the symptoms of illness can be difficult. The hope that they will go away by themselves may become a reality, but sometimes these symptoms can be the precursor of a much more serious health problem. You may try to shrug off an annoying cough which refuses to go away, a lump which you can't explain or increasingly severe discomfort which has no apparent cause. It is tempting to ignore these symptoms in the hope that they will just resolve themselves. Perhaps they can be diagnosed as a straightforward problem which can be readily sorted out – but only if you admit to the problem and consult your GP. If a more serious health issue is at stake, it is even more important to get advice and help as quickly as possible. Of course, you do not want to be heading for the surgery in a state of panic every time you sniff or sneeze, but recognizing when your body is sending messages that something more serious is afoot – and doing something about it – can make a huge difference in the longer term, as Neil discovered.

This is a period in which I do not feel any pride in my actions. I think I acted like far too many men by really making no attempt to come to terms with the changes which were obviously physically affecting me.

I had become conscious of some small but certain changes in my health but put them down to the general hassle of our everyday life running a small business and the after-effects of a personal trauma which my partner and I had suffered a month or two earlier. I further subsumed myself in work and physical activity for some bizarre reason, probably of a displacement nature. I was now swimming nearly a mile several times a week. My health was not improving and I now had some low level discomfort in my abdomen and the odd bout of nausea. This became gradually but persistently worse until I was having difficulty eating.

It was now obvious – to everybody but me – that I needed medical help. I had to be dragged the four hundred yards from home to the doctor's surgery by my partner who was determined not to leave my side until I had seen a doctor. Even then, I tried to play for time! We may have lived in the same house for eight years, but had I ever got around to registering with a GP? Why did I, a fit and healthy thirty-something man, have any need for the medical profession? So I even tried to put off this appointment by a couple of days. The doctor examined me, made a brief referral note and sketch, and instructed us to go straight to our local Accident and Emergency Unit – me, an A & E case! I think I realized then that I was about to enter the bowels of the health service and that it might be some time before I emerged again.

Whether you have a small, niggling health problem or a suspicion that it might be more serious, a cancer diagnosis is probably the last – although most feared – outcome you expect. It plunges you into a new world of blood tests and scans, physical examinations and technical terminology, fears and worries for the future. You have to get to grips with the prospect of treatment, the implications and the potential effects on your life in a very short time. It can be frightening and throw you entirely off balance at a time when you need all your reserves of strength to cope.

Fears of illness

A very real problem for many of us is overcoming the sheer, blind fear of serious illness. Not only do we have to contend with a natural fear of pain and physical debilitation but also with the much broader impact it can have on all aspects of our lives. Illness is often associated in our minds with a loss of control: your body is not behaving as it should and it is beyond your power to make it do so. We have become so accustomed to being in control of our lives, to taking decisions and mapping out our futures to suit ourselves, that any loss of control can represent a huge shock. We take for granted our ability to work or to lead an independent and active life, and if that independence is threatened then we almost inevitably feel frightened, as well as angry and perhaps cheated of something we had regarded almost as a right.

The realization that we do not have absolute control over our bodies can also have a very negative impact on the way we regard ourselves, and our self-image. Most of us define a role for ourselves and a sense of purpose in our lives, more or less consciously, in our work or other daily activities or in our personal lives as a husband, partner, father or friend. A physical threat to our ability to fulfil that role can have a very destructive effect, even causing us to question our 'usefulness'. Being unable to carry out our normal daily routine can lead to great frustration and mental debilitation.

We may also fear that illness can cause others to perceive us differently. If you have always projected an image of a strong and able man, then it can be extremely distressing to feel that others will now see you as 'weak' in some way. This fear may exist largely in your own mind rather than in the thoughts and opinions of others: you are still the same person to loved ones and friends, although you may feel that the enormity of your illness has taken over and reduced you to a relatively helpless patient.

Health awareness

Women have succeeded in recent decades in raising awareness of critical female health issues such as breast and cervical cancers, while men's health has received less attention. Screening programmes for cervical and breast cancers are now widespread and a matter of routine, in spite of the debate about the value of breast screening in terms of the whole female population. On the other hand, there is no male-specific cancer for which screening has yet been proved or accepted as valuable in the same way as cervical cancer screening has. The evidence in favour of prostate cancer screening, for example, seems also to raise difficult questions about the potential best treatment for those men who are deemed to be at risk of developing the disease.

Although 'male' cancers are now beginning to receive more publicity, men as individuals can still make an important contribution to changing attitudes by accepting the need to be aware of their own health and physical well-being.

If your car develops a puncture, then as a matter of course, you repair it as soon as possible to try to limit the damage. Similarly, if you have a health problem, serious or not, it follows that the sooner it is diagnosed, the better are your chances of successful or remedial treatment. Unfortunately, most of us feel more comfortable dealing with a car repair than with a GP about our own bodies, because there is far less at stake: it is difficult to regard health problems with any degree of objectivity.

This is not an easy obstacle to overcome, but common sense can achieve a great deal if you are prepared to listen to the signals your body is sending you. Regular testicular self-examination, for example, is encouraged in leaflets produced by the Imperial Cancer Research Fund, the Wessex Cancer Trust, the Cancer Research Campaign and Save Our Sons, to name but four organizations. However, you are unlikely to come across such information except in cancer clinics, information centres and hospitals – where few men spend any time until they are affected by cancer themselves.

Recognizing signs of change in your body is also important, but you can only achieve this if you are sufficiently self-aware to notice them. This doesn't mean that you need to subject yourself to rigorous physical examination every day, but it does mean that it is unwise to ignore your body. For example, if you are normally fit and healthy and rarely visit your doctor, but have become progressively more tired and run-down for no apparent reason, then it is sensible to consider why and to visit your GP for a check-up. Surveys have shown not only that men tend to use primary health care services less than women but also that they are more likely to delay seeking help when they become ill. It would be a mistake to think that your GP is too busy with 'more important' cases to be interested in your symptoms: if your body is behaving unusually, then you need to find out the reasons.

Most surgeries now run 'Well Man' clinics, where men of all ages can undergo a basic health check with a doctor or nurse. It is tempting to regard routine check-ups as of little value but they are a useful opportunity to remind ourselves to keep a watchful eye on our health, as well as highlighting any matters which might need our attention. The question still arises whether such screening clinics reach the sections of the population which would benefit most from their services. On the whole, they tend to be attended by the well-informed and well-motivated who are most likely to seek early help in any case if they suspect a health problem. To be of greatest value, screening needs to reach the whole population.

Some symptoms should always be treated seriously, although they will often be explained by perfectly straightforward and readily treatable conditions. You should always make an appointment to see your doctor straight away if you notice:

- unusual bleeding or discharge
- blood in stools or urine

- increased frequency in passing urine
- unusual constipation or diarrhoea
- thickening or lump in the testes
- bleeding or enlargement or changes in a mole
- other unexplained lumps
- problems in swallowing
- continuing nausea or vomiting
- continuing headaches
- persistent coughing, hoarseness or changes in the voice
- persistent abdominal discomfort or indigestion
- marked changes in weight or appetite.

Bleeding from a cut is, of course, to be expected but if you notice blood in your stools or urine or if you are coughing up blood, then you need to find out why. It may be that the bleeding is due to a bladder infection or piles or a severe chest infection, but the only way to find out is to seek medical advice. Similarly, a lump in your skin can be perfectly benign and harmless, but should nonetheless be checked by your doctor. Of course, it is easy to rationalize when faced with a potential problem: we can almost always find some explanation to fit the circumstances and a reason *not* to visit the doctor. Don't wait to see if any of these conditions clear up on their own: you have nothing to lose by seeking your GP's opinion.

Our lifestyle inevitably has an impact on our general health. We know that smoking, drinking to excess, lack of exercise and poor diet all contribute in varying measures to a whole range of health problems, from very serious diseases such as cancer to more easily rectifiable problems such as the need to lose a few pounds in weight. Lifestyle is a matter of choice in many respects and no-one can force you to adopt a 'healthy living' attitude if you choose not to. Of course, there are also factors over which you have less or no control, such as pollution in the environment or high levels of stress caused by your domestic circumstances or work.

However, as far as cancer is concerned, there are certain factors within our control which may act as triggers including:

- smoking
- excessive exposure to sunlight
- alcohol
- low-fibre, high-fat diet.

It would not be practical or realistic to base our lives around the impact of our every action on our chances of developing cancer. We take calculated risks in many ways every day, from crossing the road to eating certain foods. But we should at least be aware of the risks we are running, and aware of the possible consequences.

2
Cancer

One of the keys to coping with any difficult situation is to have sufficient information and knowledge of the facts to enable you to understand what you are facing and to make reasonably well-informed decisions. The first problem for most men when faced with a diagnosis of cancer is a very sketchy knowledge of what cancer is. Even if you have had previous contact with someone who has been treated for cancer, there is a high chance that you knew only a little about their condition. Knowledge is very important, because it gives you the power to take a more active role in the management of your disease – if you want to.

How much you decide to find out about your cancer is entirely dependent on you. Some people like to be told or read quite detailed technical information about their cancer. Others prefer to know only as much as they are told by their doctors and oncologists (specialist cancer doctors) and choose not to ask for more indepth information. In any case, a basic understanding of how cancer develops and some detail about your own cancer in particular will be of benefit to you and those close to you, if not at the beginning of your journey through treatment, then almost certainly later on.

This chapter looks at cancer in two ways:

- general information about how cancer develops
- information about specific cancers.

What is cancer?

The body is made up of cells which are continually multiplying and working to replace those which have become damaged or worn out. This is a constant process which keeps the body working normally and 'repairs' it when, for example, you suffer an injury or have an operation. Cells in different parts of the body have different life cycles and multiply at different rates, but what is common to them all is that they contain signals which tell them how to behave and when to multiply.

11

Cancer happens when a single normal cell starts behaving abnormally. The cell begins to divide and grow uncontrollably because the signals which tell it how to behave are not working properly. The same happens to the cells it produces but because these cells are so minute, the effect of their growth can remain undetected in the body at this stage. The place in the body where this abnormal growth begins is known as the primary site of the cancer and the resulting tumour as the primary tumour. Although there are many, many different cancers, they are generally described in terms of their site of origin, so that lung cancer refers to a tumour which originated in the lung.

The next stage in the development of the cancer is for the cells to invade the tissue which immediately surrounds them. Next they can circulate to other parts of the body via the bloodstream or lymph vessels, which both reach all parts of the body and therefore provide an easy means of 'transport' for the cancer cells. The cancer cells arrive at a new site in the body (which can be quite distant from the primary tumour) and again invade the surrounding tissue. The resulting tumour is known as a secondary tumour or metastasis, and is directly related to the primary tumour. For example, bowel cancer tends to spread via the vascular system to the liver. The secondary tumour in the liver is not referred to as cancer of the liver, but as a 'secondary cancer of the bowel'. The distinction is important in understanding your cancer: in this example, the spread does *not* mean that you are suffering from cancer of the bowel *and* cancer of the liver. It is the ability of the cancer cells to travel around the body and invade other sites which makes cancer such a difficult disease to treat effectively. If it were simply a question of treating a single abnormal 'lump', then this could in many cases be removed surgically and the problem eliminated.

Different cancers spread and invade other sites in the body at varying rates, but the sites where they metastasize (form secondary cancers) tend to follow a pattern. For example, testicular cancer spreads first to the lymph nodes in the abdomen, sometimes to the lungs and in some cases to the liver or brain.

Although cancers are generally described by their site of origin, you may also encounter other terms used to describe your cancer, according to the type of tissue where it originated. The most common of these are:

Carcinoma

Carcinomas account for a large proportion of all cancers. A carcinoma is a cancer which originates in the epithelial cells of the body. This is a layer of lining or covering cells which is found in the lungs, the stomach and digestive system and also on the surface of the skin and in glands throughout the body.

Sarcoma

Sarcomas are less common. A sarcoma is a cancer which forms in the tissues which connect the parts of the body together – the bones, muscle, cartilage, tendon and so on.

Lymphoma

Lymphoma refers to the cancers which originate in the lymph nodes and lymphatic tissue, although some lymphomas can start in the bone marrow.

Leukaemia

Leukaemias are cancers of blood cells. They originate in the bone marrow and affect the white cells in the blood and, in turn, also the red cells. The white cells are important because they affect your body's ability to fight infection and the red cells carry oxygen around the body.

A relatively small number of different cancers account for a high proportion of cases newly registered each year, the more common being the lung, colorectal, prostate and bladder cancers. These account for around half of the total cases and, as with many cancers, are most common in older men. The main exceptions to this for men are cancer of the testis whose incidence peaks before the age of 40, and the leukaemias which have two peaks, one before the age of 20 and the other around the age of 70.

Learning more about your cancer

Your own doctor or oncologist is the best person to answer detailed questions about your specific cancer. However, it can be very difficult to absorb medical information which is given to you verbally when you are feeling vulnerable and possibly very unwell. This section provides some basic details of the more common cancers which affect men, by their site of origin.

It looks first at the male-specific cancers which, by definition, affect only men and cannot affect women. Although they are not necessarily the cancers which affect the largest numbers of men (these are traditionally the lung and bowel cancers), they are the cancers for which men need to have an especial awareness, in the same way that women are especially aware of breast and cervical cancers. The other cancers included in this section are those which are statistically most prevalent amongst the male population. The different cancers are covered in the following order:

- prostate cancer
- testicular cancer
- lung cancer
- non-melanoma skin cancers
- cancer of the urinary tract – kidney and bladder
- cancer of the bowel – colon and rectum
- stomach cancer
- non-Hodgkin's lymphoma
- leukaemias

Please remember throughout this section that the facts given are necessarily brief and generalized and are intended to provide you with a first step towards understanding more about your cancer. Your doctor and oncologist will be able to give you more detailed information about your cancer and recommend further books or leaflets for you to read in your own time, if you feel this would be helpful. The British Association of Cancer United Patients (BACUP – tel: 0800 181 199 and 0171 613 2121) publishes a series of booklets on different cancers, treatments and related topics. These are available free to people with cancer. *Don't be afraid to ask* if you ever feel you need more information.

The mainstream cancer treatments, which are by necessity mentioned here in relation to each of the cancers discussed, are covered in detail in Chapter 3.

A glossary of the more common medical terms which you may encounter is included at the end of the book.

Prostate cancer

This is one of the specifically male cancers about which there has been most publicity in recent years. There has been debate about whether men should be routinely screened for prostate cancer, although so far no action has been taken to put this into effect. It is a cancer which rarely affects younger men. However, age is a very significant factor in determining the nature of treatment: it is usually only younger men for whom radical surgery is appropriate as potentially curative treatment. This does *not* mean that older men will not receive effective treatment!

Why is age so important in prostate cancer? If you are an older man for whom prostate cancer has been diagnosed, it may seem very 'ageist' and unjust that the most radical treatments are usually proposed only for younger men. However, the majority of men with prostate cancer actually die from causes *other than* their cancer: they die 'with' their cancer, not 'from' it. This is why it is the men who develop prostate cancer at a younger age for whom it is more likely to be life-threatening, and therefore for whom curative treatment (treatment which is intended to bring about a complete cure) rather than palliative treatment (treatment which will alleviate the symptoms of cancer without the intention to cure it) is most appropriate.

It should be stressed that the symptoms of prostate cancer are the same as those for enlargement of the prostate, which is experienced by many men over the age of about sixty. Experiencing these symptoms is *not* necessarily an indication that you are suffering from prostate cancer, although it would be wise to seek your doctor's advice.

The symptoms you might notice include

- difficulty or 'hesitancy' in beginning to urinate
- unusual frequency of urination
- unusual urgency in needing to urinate
- unexplained pain in the lower back or abdomen
- 'dribbling' at the end of urination.

In most cases, cancer of the prostate grows slowly and most men with prostate cancer die of something else first. The prostate is a small gland situated beneath the bladder and in front of the rectum and in most men it becomes larger with increasing age. It is worth stressing again that enlargement of the prostate does *not* mean that cancer will necessarily develop.

Diagnosis is made by means of rectal examination, blood tests for tumour markers (see glossary) and a biopsy in which a small piece of prostate tissue is examined to see if there is any cancer present.

Depending on the results of the initial tests, X-rays and scans may be carried out to determine whether any spread to other parts of the body has occurred. The site to which prostate cancer tends to spread most commonly is the lymph nodes in the pelvis, although the bones and rarely the liver can be affected.

The type of treatment used depends on whether the cancer has spread beyond the prostate gland and your age at the time of diagnosis. If the cancer has not spread and you are aged up to about 60, then radical surgery to remove the gland may be considered. One of the side effects of the operation can be impotence, so it is important to discuss it carefully and in detail with your specialist and your spouse or partner to make sure that you are fully aware of the implications before surgery is undertaken. If it is felt that surgery is not appropriate, then prostate cancer can also be treated with radiotherapy. Again, there is a risk of impotence and this and other side effects need to be fully understood before the treatment is undertaken. In some cases, careful monitoring might be chosen as a preferable form of treatment. This might be appropriate if the cancer is very slow growing and has not spread outside the prostate, and if there are other health considerations (including age) which make the other options less advisable.

When discussing forms of treatment with your doctors, it is very important for you to be aware of whether the intention of treatment is curative or palliative (as distinguished in Chapters 3 and 4). This is not *necessarily* because palliative treatment is a second-best option, but because it is important for your own understanding of your cancer.

If the cancer has spread, then the treatment proposed will be different to take account of this factor. Hormone therapy is one option. Prostate cancer often needs male hormones for its growth (mostly testosterone), so hormone therapy which stifles the supply of male hormone can be effective. This is usually achieved in one of two ways

- by using drugs which block the release or action of male hormones – which may cause impotence;
- by surgical removal of the testes.

Again, you need to discuss with your specialist which option is most appropriate in your case, and weigh up the pros and cons of each treatment. In addition, radiotherapy can be given and directed at the area of the body to which the cancer has spread. Chemotherapy is only rarely used for prostate cancer at present.

Testicular cancer

Testicular cancer is one of the rarer forms of cancer and is unusual in that it tends to occur at a relatively young age; it reaches its peak, statistically, between the ages of 25 and 35. Although the total number of men diagnosed with testicular cancer is comparatively low, it is the most common form of cancer for younger men in the 20 to 40 age group. It also has an extremely high cure rate, particularly if it is diagnosed in its early stages, but there is also a good chance of a cure even if it has spread.

There are two main types of testicular cancer – seminomas and teratomas. Seminomas are slower growing and spread to the lymph nodes in the abdomen. The teratomas also spread to these lymph nodes and have a greater tendency to spread elsewhere in the body, particularly to the lungs and sometimes to the liver or brain.

The most common sign of testicular cancer is a lump on the testicle, which is often painless, and in some cases it may be very small and go unnoticed for some time. For this reason, it is extremely important for all men to check their testicles regularly for any abnormalities. Other symptoms include back pain, and shortness of breath if the cancer has spread to the lungs.

The first step in diagnosis is the surgical removal of the testicular lump and the affected testicle. The lump is examined under a microscope to establish whether the cancer is a seminoma or teratoma: this is important as the two types require different treatments. Your blood will be tested for the presence of tumour markers called alpha-fetoprotein, beta human chorionic gonadotrophin and placental alkaline phosphatase. These markers (often referred to as AFP, BhCG and PLAP respectively) are very reliable indicators of the level of cancer present, and will be used later in monitoring your progress. You will also have X-rays and scans to determine whether the cancer has spread elsewhere in your body. If the cancer has been diagnosed at an early stage and there is no evidence of spread, then there may be no need for treatment other than surgery, although you will be actively monitored for a considerable time. Your blood will be tested for tumour markers and you will have scans to detect any recurrence for at least two years.

In the case of seminomas with or without spread to other parts of the body, the next step in treatment may be radiotherapy, although in some cases chemotherapy might be considered. For teratomas where the cancer has spread to other parts of the body, chemotherapy is used. In both cases, the aim of treatment is a cure and the amount of treatment given will depend upon the extent of the spread of cancer. With teratomas, some residual scar tissue often remains in the abdomen after treatment is completed. Surgery may well be proposed to remove the residual tissue in order to determine whether it still contains any cancerous cells.

After treatment is completed, you will have regular check-ups for some years, with blood tests and scans to check that there is no recurrence. Even if the cancer recurs later, there is still a good chance of a cure in many cases.

As testicular cancer tends to affect younger men, another very important point to be considered at an early stage is the possibility of sperm banking, as the treatment may make you infertile. Sperm banking must be done before treatment starts, so it is important to discuss it as soon as possible with your doctors. Unfortunately, some men with testicular cancer have a low sperm count even before treatment starts, so their sperm may not be suitable for banking. In some men – and depending on the treatment proposed – fertility may return after a year or two.

Lung cancer

The main symptoms of lung cancer are

- shortness of breath
- chronic cough, sometimes with blood in the sputum
- chest pain and/or infection

Most lung cancers originate in the air tubes in the lungs, and can be split into two main categories – non-small cell tumours and small cell tumours.

In diagnosing both small cell and non-small cell lung cancer, tests will be performed to establish the extent of any spread. These may involve a combination of blood tests, X-rays and scans, and an examination of the lungs and lymph nodes in the chest by using a thin telescope. This is either inserted via the mouth to look at the lungs (bronchoscope) or via a small incision in the neck (mediastino-scope) under anaesthetic to examine the lymph nodes.

Non-small cell tumours usually grow more slowly although their prognosis is still not good, and often follow a pattern of spreading first to the lymph nodes in the chest and neck, and later to the liver, bone and brain. If the tumour is small and accessible and has not yet spread to the lymph nodes, then surgical removal may be possible. The other most common form of treatment is radiotherapy. Although it is not usually curative, it can help by relieving blockage by the tumour of major airways, and by reducing pain.

Small cell tumours generally spread faster and thus frequently involve multiple parts of the body, even before they are diagnosed. The areas affected tend to be the liver, bone marrow and brain. For this type of tumour, chemotherapy is the most effective form of treatment, to which radiotherapy may be added because if the cancer has already spread then surgically removing the primary tumour in the lung will not have any effect on the secondary tumours.

Non-melanoma skin cancers

Non-melanoma skin cancers are common and in many cases completely curable. They are often associated with prolonged exposure to harsh sunlight, and in particular to ultraviolet rays, and are more of a risk to fair-skinned people. These cancers are divided into two categories, basal cell cancer and squamous cell cancer.

Basal cell skin cancer (also known as rodent ulcers) is usually slow growing, and almost never spreads elsewhere in the body. The main symptom you might notice is a whitish sore on the skin which becomes ulcerated. Squamous cell skin cancer is less common and is slightly more likely to spread to other sites in the body. It can appear on parts of the skin which have previously suffered damage, and is characterized by a hard, red and scaly area. Both types rarely cause any bleeding until a later stage in their development.

The diagnosis is usually made by biopsy, with possible further examination to check for any spread.

Treatment by surgery is usually possible, and depending on how aggressive the tumour is and whether it has spread, it often results in a cure. In some cases, electrosurgery (cauterization) or cryosurgery might be used, which use heat and freezing respectively to remove small tumours. If the site of the tumour is such that surgery would be difficult with a smaller chance of a good result, radiotherapy can be used, and also has very good cure rates.

Urinary tract cancers

Bladder cancer

Bladder cancer is roughly twice as prevalent in men as in women and, as with prostate cancer, it is more likely to occur with increasing age. It is believed to be more common in people who smoke, as the chemical products of smoking travel via the lungs and bloodstream into the bladder before being passed out of the body. It is also more common in those who have worked in the dye or rubber industries.

Bladder cancer can be non-invasive or invasive. The non-invasive form does not grow deep into the wall of the bladder. The invasive form can cover a large area of the inner surface of the bladder as well as invading deeper into the bladder wall. If this occurs, the cancer can also spread to the lymph nodes and later progress to distant sites such as the lungs, liver and bones.

The symptom you are most likely to notice is blood in your urine (haematuria). You may also be aware of a need to pass urine more often than usual and experience discomfort or pain on passing urine (dysuria). It's important to remember that both symptoms can often be caused by a non-cancerous problem – such as a readily treatable infection – but this is no reason to delay a check-up with your doctor.

You will undergo various tests to establish whether cancer is present, and these may include urine tests and an internal examination of the bladder with a cystoscope. This is a means of looking inside the bladder with a thin tube containing a type of telescope and may be done under either general or local anaesthetic. You may also have X-rays and scans of the kidneys, abdomen and the pelvis.

The treatment for the non-invasive type of bladder cancer involves cystoscopy, with cauterization or removal by laser of any tumour and then regular follow-up cystoscopy. Drugs may also be instilled into the bladder. The more invasive type of cancer may involve more extensive surgery, possibly with the removal of the whole bladder (cystectomy). This also involves the requirement to reconstruct the bladder or to divert the flow of urine, and you will need to discuss this in detail with your doctors so that you fully understand the impact that the surgery will have on your life. Radiotherapy may be an option to consider instead of surgery, but this will depend upon your particular circumstances. Chemotherapy may be proposed. Although its role is not yet fully defined, bladder cancer (including secondary disease) can respond well to chemotherapy.

Kidney cancer

Kidney cancer tends to be slightly more prevalent in men than in women, and there appears to be a similar link with smoking. The kidneys act as a hugely powerful filter of the blood, separating the 'good' elements which are needed by the body from the waste, which is passed out of the body as urine. The kidneys are extremely efficient and although we have two, the body could manage perfectly well with only one.

The main type of kidney cancer is renal-cell carcinoma. Its main symptoms are bleeding, which will be noticed in the urine, and possibly pain, discomfort or swelling in the kidney region – in your back and side of the abdomen, below the ribs. Again, it should be stressed that blood in your urine may result from a cause other than cancer, but it should nonetheless warrant an appointment with your doctor.

Kidney cancer can spread via the lymph nodes, but may also travel to other parts of the body via the bloodstream. Diagnosis is likely to involve physical examination, urine tests and various X-rays (with dyes to show unusual features in the kidney), and scans to check whether the cancer has spread.

Surgery is generally the mainstay of treatment in kidney cancer. Treatment is likely to involve surgery to remove the affected kidney, sometimes even when the cancer has spread further. If it has not spread, then the hope is for a complete cure. Even if it has spread, the surgery can be worthwhile to relieve any pain and discomfort.

Other therapies might be proposed, such as hormone therapy or chemotherapy, and if so these should be discussed with your doctors.

Bowel cancer – colon and rectum

Cancers of the colon and rectum are amongst the most common cancers. They tend to progress relatively slowly, and usually follow the same pattern of spread from the inside of the bowel, through its wall and via veins and lymph nodes to the liver and/or lungs.

There has been much debate about the contribution of diet to the development of bowel cancers, and it is thought that too much saturated fat and too little fibre do increase the risk of bowel cancer. Your bowel habit can play a role: chronic constipation can be a contributory factor to bowel cancer. Family history is a very important factor in some cases.

Cancer of the bowel can be difficult to detect in its early stages, as the warning signs can be easily overlooked. The symptoms you may notice include blood in your stools, a change in your bowel habit to diarrhoea or constipation and abdominal pain and swelling. Blood in your stool can, of course, be caused by other conditions such as haemorrhoids – but you should still consult your doctor to check.

The diagnosis of bowel cancer involves physical examination, testing of the stool to check whether blood is present, a barium enema X-ray to look at the bowel in more detail and usually further scans to check whether any spread has occurred.

Surgery forms a major part of treatment for cancer of the bowel. Since the aim is to remove the tumour completely this may involve removing a significant portion of the bowel itself, depending on the size and position of the tumour. This may lead to a need for a temporary or permanent colostomy or ileostomy (these are discussed in Chapter 3), so it is very important to discuss the extent and nature of surgery in detail with your doctor to ensure that you fully understand the likely results and implications. If the cancer is still in its early stages, then surgery may bring a complete cure – although it will be some years before this can be confirmed. Radiotherapy may also be considered, usually in addition to surgery as a follow-up treatment, as may chemotherapy.

Stomach cancer

Stomach cancer is another of the cancers which tends to be roughly twice as prevalent in men than in women. It can behave in different ways, depending on whether it is of a more superficial and less aggressive type or more invasive and aggressive. It begins in the stomach lining, and can spread through the stomach wall from where it is able to start invading nearby lymph nodes and other organs such as the pancreas and spleen. It may also spread to the liver via the bloodstream.

It is clear that there are links between the incidence of stomach cancer and some types of diet.

One of the problems with stomach cancer is that it may not produce any readily distinguishable symptoms in its early stages. Signs which you may become aware of include an indigestion-type ache, pain in the upper part of the abdomen and a general sense of tiredness, loss of appetite and weight loss. These are, of course, symptoms which many of us experience from time to time and to which we may therefore attach little significance. If they persist, however, then you should have a check-up with your doctor.

Diagnosis of stomach cancer is by taking a biopsy, which is done using a gastroscope, a tube which is passed into the stomach via the mouth to look at the stomach and take samples. You are also likely to have a barium meal X-ray of your stomach, in which the barium you drink is highlighted on the X-ray and makes it easier for doctors to examine the contents of your stomach. You may also have blood tests and further scans, to check whether there is any spread of cancer.

Surgery is the main form of treatment for stomach cancer and the details of the operation will depend upon the location of the tumour and whether the cancer has spread. Radiotherapy may be used if surgery is not feasible or to control symptoms if the tumour has spread beyond the stomach. Chemotherapy may be useful in some cases, particularly for the relief of symptoms when the cancer has spread.

Non-Hodgkin's lymphomas

Lymphomas are a group of cancers which start in the lymphatic system and usually spread via the lymph nodes which are situated in the neck, armpits, the middle of the chest and in the abdomen. Some lymphomas are slow-growing (low grade) and others progress very quickly (high grade): if untreated the latter can cause serious problems within a few months. Others fall somewhere between the two extremes. The lymphomas generally start in the lymph nodes, and may also involve the bone marrow depending on how aggressive the cancer is. High grade non-Hodgkin's lymphoma is often completely curable.

Symptoms you might notice include a painless but persistent

23

swelling in your lymph nodes, usually in the neck, armpit or groin. In fact, enlarged lymph nodes often result from straightforward viral infections and are very common – but these clear up within a few weeks. Enlarged lymph nodes which are not accompanied by any infection, which do not disappear on their own and which are not tender to the touch, should be regarded seriously and checked by your doctor. Of course, there may be a perfectly innocent cause but the check-up can do you no harm. More general symptoms which tend to accompany lymphoma as it progresses are a general tiredness, loss of appetite and of weight and unusual sweating at night.

Lymphoma is usually diagnosed by means of a biopsy of the enlarged lymph node, which will help to determine the type of lymphoma in question: there are several dozen and the classification of lymphoma is a very complex area. Once the type of lymphoma is established, further tests will be carried out to establish how far it has spread and these may include a chest X-ray, lymphogram and scans. Both the type and spread of a lymphoma are important factors in determining the nature and extent of treatment you will undergo.

If your lymphoma is the slow-growing, low-grade type, then you may experience periods of time where no treatment at all is considered necessary. However, you are likely to undergo some chemotherapy at certain stages to keep the effects and symptoms of your cancer manageable – and this type of treatment may last for some years. In some cases, radiotherapy might be helpful to relieve problems if an enlarged lymph node is, for example, blocking another organ and causing trouble.

Treatment for the higher grades of lymphoma differs in that the cancer is faster and more steadily growing, and therefore cannot be left untreated for periods of time as the lower-grade lymphomas can. Chemotherapy is commonly used and it can lead to a cure. Radiotherapy may be used at the same time to treat localized areas of tumour.

Leukaemias

The group of leukaemias is divided into categories depending on where they originate and whether they are fast or slow growing. They all affect the cells which are produced in the bone marrow (and/or the lymph nodes) which then form the red and white blood cells. There are four main types of leukaemia:

- chronic lymphocytic leukaemia (CLL) is a slow growing cancer of one type of white cell, the lymphocytes;
- chronic granulocytic (or myeloid) leukaemia (CGL or CML) is a slow growing cancer of another type of white cell, the granulocytes;
- acute lymphoblastic leukaemia (ALL) is a faster growing cancer of the lymphocytes;
- acute myeloid leukaemia (AML) is a faster growing cancer of the granulocytes.

The lymphocytes and granulocytes are different types of white cell whose purpose is to help the body to fight infection. If your white cells are not working efficiently, then your body will have difficulty fighting off infections. The more acute forms of leukaemia produce very immature white cells which can be identified in the bloodstream.

It is important to be aware that the words 'chronic' and 'acute' refer to how quickly the cancer grows, not to how 'bad' the cancer is. Chronic types tend to affect adults more than children, and acute types children more than adults.

Chronic leukaemias may produce no symptoms at all for some time, as they are slow growing. All of the leukaemias are likely to be diagnosed by a blood test and possibly a bone marrow sample, with additional tests such as X-rays and scans to check whether any other organs are affected.

Chemotherapy is the mainstay of treatment in leukaemias. The type varies from simple tablets up to and including a requirement for bone marrow transplantation in some cases. Bone marrow transplantation is a very gruelling treatment, however, and your general medical condition will be important in deciding whether the benefits of the treatment outweigh the risks. Additionally, in some cases, chemicals need to be injected around the spinal cord and radiotherapy given to the brain.

3

Cancer treatments

The prospect of embarking upon a journey through cancer treatment is often made more difficult because we have little knowledge about how it works and what it 'looks like'. This can contribute to a sense of fear and trepidation, because it is a journey into the unknown. Before you start any treatment, your doctors will explain the planned course of action to you but it is still natural to feel daunted, not least because you are still trying to come to terms with your cancer diagnosis and the changes this has brought to your life. Don't ever feel afraid to ask doctors or nurses questions or to repeat explanations to you if you feel you haven't fully grasped or absorbed what they have told you. It is very important that you come to understand the nature of your treatment and the potential outcome.

Although progress is being made in newer therapies, the most common treatments for cancer are

- surgery
- radiotherapy
- chemotherapy.

The intent behind treatment can be 'curative' or 'palliative'. Treatment whose intent is curative aims to cure a patient completely of his cancer, so that no evidence of it remains and he returns to normal health. A cure means that all evidence of your cancer is eliminated and that it will not return. However, the term 'cure' can only be applied with confidence after the passage of time – in the majority of cases, after five years. 'Palliative' treatment does not aim to cure, but the term can be used in two different contexts. First, palliative treatment can be used to shrink a tumour and thereby improve the patient's quality of life. This does not necessarily mean that you have only a short time to live, but rather that it is not thought possible to eradicate your cancer completely: for example, the majority of men with prostate cancer actually die from something other than their cancer. Second, palliative care may be used purely to control and alleviate the symptoms of cancer where no other treatment options are available. It is important for you to clarify with your doctor the intent behind your treatment. This may be a difficult question to ask, and indeed a difficult question for your doctor to answer, but you will be better prepared to cope with your treatment if you understand what it is intended to achieve. The terms such as 'cure' or 'remission' which your doctors may use in discussing the intent behind your treatment are described in more detail in Chapter 4.

A tremendous amount of research has been carried out in recent decades to establish the most effective type of treatment for individual cancers. Just as there are several hundred different forms of the disease, so there are many ways in which treatment can be geared to your particular cancer. Different cancers behave and react in different ways, so the appropriate treatment for, say, bowel cancer will not be the same as the treatment for lung cancer. You may have a single type of treatment or a combination of treatments, say, surgery followed by chemotherapy or radiotherapy, but you can be assured that the decision as to which is most appropriate for you will be based on the most effective proven treatment for your particular circumstances.

Once your cancer has been diagnosed, treatment often starts very quickly and it is easy to feel that you are being carried along by events beyond your control and understanding. Finding out as much as you can about your proposed treatment and, just as importantly, about any anticipated side-effects, can help you to regain some sense of control. Building up knowledge does take time, especially in such difficult circumstances, but knowing what to expect will help you to cope better once the treatment is underway.

Surgery

Why is surgery needed?

Surgery remains an important element in the treatment of many cancers and it may be proposed for several reasons:

- to remove the primary tumour entirely and thereby establish a diagnosis;
- to remove as much cancerous tissue as possible before proceeding to other forms of treatment;
- to alleviate symptoms or the effects of your cancer, such as a bowel obstruction, even if surgery is not the main form of treatment.

27

There are some types of cancer such as leukaemias and lymphomas for which surgery is not appropriate because the cancer is, by definition, not restricted to a localized and operable site in the body.

While surgery may be helpful in many cases, there are circumstances where an operation is not a practical option. This may be because it is felt that the risk to you as the patient would be too great or because it would not be possible to remove enough of the tumour to make surgery the most effective treatment at this stage. This might be the case if your cancer has already spread, making cure by surgery alone impossible, while the lump itself is not causing you problems. It does not necessarily mean that surgery is completely ruled out later, but rather that alternative forms of treatment are felt to be more appropriate at this stage. It is worth reiterating that your doctors will propose the treatment which they feel is likely to be most effective for your particular circumstances.

What will surgery entail?

If the cancer is confined to a localized site, it may be possible to remove the diseased tissue surgically, together with part or all of the affected body organ. If the cancer has spread to other sites in the body, then it is more likely that either surgery will not be recommended at all, with the focus on treating the whole body, or the surgery will be designed to remove the primary tumour (the 'source' of the cancer) before using other forms of therapy to treat the secondary cancer. In all cases, the decision to operate will depend upon where your cancer is situated and whether your oncologist and surgeon feel it is safe and reasonable to operate on it. Before surgery goes ahead, tests and scans will be carried out to build up as detailed a picture as possible about your cancer, but it is obviously not possible for a surgeon to assess exactly what will be found once the operation is underway.

Some forms of surgery are obviously more complex and invasive than others: an operation for melanoma (skin cancer) differs greatly from surgery for cancer of the bowel. It is therefore very important to discuss your operation in advance, and to be clear about the possible implications. By definition, surgery involves some degree of physical damage to the body. This may be limited to an inconspicuous scar which will fade in time and cause no long-term distress, but in some cases the damage will be more severe. There may be more obvious physical impairment, which can be difficult to accept at first, such as the removal of a testicle in cases of testicular cancer. We are all concerned to some degree by physical appearances, and if your operation will necessarily cause some change to the appearance or behaviour of your body then it is important to understand this in advance. For example, it may be possible to insert a prosthesis in cases where a testicle has been removed. Sometimes the consequences of surgery will have a more far-reaching effect on your life.

For example, one of the possible outcomes of surgery for certain types of cancer, where part of the bowel or bladder is removed, is that the body can no longer deal with its waste products in the normal way, either temporarily or permanently. To allow the body to get rid of its waste, the surgeon has to create a 'stoma', a small opening on the surface of the abdomen. There are three types of stoma:

- a colostomy is a stoma in the large bowel (colon);
- an ileostomy is a stoma in part of the small bowel (ileum);
- a urostomy is a stoma in the urinary system.

A stoma is created during the operation. The surgeon will bring a healthy part of your colon, ileum or urinary system to the new opening on the surface of the skin. A bag is attached to the opening into which the bowel or bladder contents can pass.

This procedure will only be necessary in certain specific cases. However, if there is a possibility that it is needed, it is very important to discuss it in advance so that you have the opportunity to prepare yourself for its effects. The prospect of living with a stoma can be distressing at first, but the majority of stoma patients can manage to adapt so that their lives are as near normal as possible. You will be taught how to empty and look after your bag, so that it becomes a normal part of your daily routine. A stoma nurse will be able to talk to you about your stoma and advise you about, for example, dietary considerations or any fears you may have about its effect on your life and how you can best cope.

If your operation will have specific effects on your life in the future, you may need extra support and information about how best to adapt and cope. The medical team attached to the ward where you have your surgery will be experienced in helping patients come to terms with these changes, and it makes sense to draw on their knowledge and expertise and to ask them how other people cope best. Many specialist wards also keep a range of leaflets dealing with the particular issues their patients are likely to face. If these are not obviously available then do ask, or approach your GP if you prefer.

Are there any alternatives to surgery?

The very nature of surgery can make it a frightening prospect, and you may wonder whether less invasive alternatives exist to treat your cancer. This is very much a matter for consideration on a case by case basis, and should be discussed with your team of doctors. Surgery will not be recommended without good and specific reasons. If alternative treatments are available for your type of cancer, then these will be explained to you and the relative chances of a successful outcome assessed. The final choice to have surgery or not will always be yours, but based on as much information as you wish to be given.

Coping with surgery

Before you undergo surgery, it is important to understand not only the physical nature of the operation, but also its more general effects. You may need to make arrangements for extra support and care while you are convalescing, for example, or to let your employer know for how long you may be unable to work. It can be useful to prepare a list of questions to ask the surgeon when you meet him or her and to have a member of your family or a close friend with you for extra support. The idea of a list of questions may seem over-formal, but it is very easy to forget issues which are important to you when you are feeling worried and possibly very unwell. They might include:

- How long will I be in hospital? This will depend both on the type of operation and on your own physical state: a young, basically fit young man may recover more quickly than someone older and in less good general health.
- How long will I be convalescent? Again, this varies between individuals, but you will cope more easily and be in a better position to make appropriate arrangements if you know that you will need more help and support than usual for, say, a week or a fortnight or a month.

- How much pain or discomfort should I expect, and what sort of pain relief will be provided?
- What can I expect when I wake after the operation?
- How much scarring will there be?
- What other physical effects can I expect?
- Will there be any impairment of my sexual function?
- What sort of post-operative follow-up will there be? (check-up by your surgeon, further tests, X-rays or scans, etc). How soon?
- What will happen next? (additional chemotherapy or radiotherapy treatment, monitoring, etc).
- Who will perform the operation?

Surgery is necessarily an invasive procedure and it is natural to have qualms about agreeing to an operation. If you are as well-prepared for it as possible by talking it over beforehand, then you are likely to find its effects easier to cope with afterwards.

Radiotherapy

Most of us are familiar with the use of radiation in X-rays. In much higher doses it can be effective in treating certain cancers by damaging and in some cases completely destroying the cancerous tissue. It also has an important role in palliative care, as it can help to relieve some symptoms of cancer such as pain and bleeding.

The aim of curative radiotherapy treatment is to direct a very carefully measured dose of radiation to the area of the tumour and thereby to kill off the cancerous cells. The dose needs to be high enough to shrink the tumour but not so high that it also damages the surrounding normal, healthy tissue, which may be affected in the short term but should be able to repair itself in time. Some cancers respond very well to radiotherapy, and in some cases it may be sufficient to effect a cure.

Radiotherapy may also be used to shrink a tumour prior to an operation to surgically remove it, the aim being to make the surgeon's job more straightforward. It has an important role, too, in cancers where surgery would not be possible.

There are two basic types of radiotherapy: external and internal. In neither type will you become permanently radioactive and, in the external type, you will not actually be in contact with radioactivity at any point.

It is most common for radiotherapy to be administered externally, by directing radiation at the tumour site using a radiotherapy machine, which looks very much like an X-ray machine. However, for some cancers radiotherapy is given internally, by temporarily placing a radioactive source either in or next to the tumour. Sometimes, it may be given in the form of a radioactive drink.

External radiotherapy

Radiotherapy is often given as an out-patient, if you are well enough to be at home and to travel each day to the hospital.

Planning is a very important part of radiotherapy treatment, to ensure that you receive the appropriate dose of radiation and that it is directed at exactly the right points on your body. Scans and X-rays will help your doctors to plan your treatment as these will assist doctors to establish the exact size and position of your tumour. Ink marks may be made on your skin where the radiation is to be directed, or if you are having radiotherapy to your head or neck region, then a see-through mould of the area may be constructed to keep your head absolutely still, and the ink markings will be made on this mould. The planning stage of your treatment may take some time and is likely to occupy the whole of your first appointment. It is tempting to feel impatient and natural to want to start the treatment as soon as possible. However, precise and careful planning is a vital stage of your treatment and cannot be rushed.

The dose of radiation you are to receive will be calculated precisely. It will then be split up into a number of smaller doses or 'fractions' which you will receive over a period of days or weeks, usually on Monday to Friday, with a recovery period at the weekend. The strength and number of doses will be tailored to your specific circumstances – your type of cancer and how advanced it is, and your general state of health must all be taken into consideration.

Various machines may be used to administer radiotherapy, either from one or more fixed positions or while rotating around your body. Before you have your treatment, you will be positioned very carefully by the radiographers so that the radiation is directed at exactly the right point. You may feel awkward if you have to hold a slightly uncomfortable position, but the treatment itself is painless and will take between a few seconds and a few minutes. In fact, many people are surprised at how quickly the radiation treatment itself is administered.

Internal radiotherapy – caesium or iridium implants

If you are having internal radiotherapy, you will stay in hospital for your treatment. A fine needle, wire or tube carrying the radioactive 'source' is placed into or next to the cancerous tissue under general anaesthetic, and remains in place until you have received the appropriate dose of radiation. After you have had the correct dose, which is tailored precisely to your particular circumstances, the implant is removed. The intention of the treatment is to administer the radiation to the cancerous tissue while causing as little damage as possible to the healthy tissue which surrounds it.

While you are having your treatment, the hospital will take precautions to avoid the possibility of exposing either your visitors or the staff who are caring for you to radiation. You will probably be nursed in a side room, and lead screens may be placed around your bed to absorb any radiation given out. Nurses and doctors will only spend short periods at a time in your room, and your visitors may be restricted to short visits or asked to talk to you from outside.

These precautions may seem rather severe at a time when you need the support of family and friends more than usual. However, they should only be necessary for a short period, and only while your radioactive implant is in place. You may find it helps to distract yourself as much as possible by watching TV, reading or listening to the radio, for example. This may not be easy when you are worried and feeling under stress, but it is worth persevering as it will help to make your time in hospital pass more quickly.

Some people worry about the continuing risk of radiation after the treatment is over. Once the radioactive implant is removed, all radiation disappears. If your treatment is in the form of a radioactive liquid, then you may have to wait for some days for the radioactivity to lessen before you can leave. You and your belongings will be checked thoroughly to check you are free of radioactivity, and you will be advised of any precautions you should follow when you get home.

Side-effects

The aim of radiotherapy is to destroy the cancer cells, but it can also affect the surrounding healthy tissue, and you may experience some side-effects as a result. Different people react in different ways to their treatment so it will not be possible to predict exactly how you will be affected, but your doctors will try to make sure that you are as well-prepared as possible. Side-effects can be split into two categories, those which are general and those which depend on the area of your body which is being treated.

The more common general side-effects include:

- Feeling more tired than usual, which may be compounded by the need to travel to and from the hospital every day. Don't be afraid to rest more than usual: if you need to take a nap in the afternoon, then do so.
- Nausea and possibly vomiting, although this depends to some degree on the strength and number of doses of radiotherapy. If this is a problem, you will be given anti-sickness drugs which are generally very effective. This tends to occur more when any area of the bowel or certain areas of the brain are in the radiation field.
- A skin reaction similar to sunburn may develop. The staff treating you will advise you about skin care during your treatment.
- Weight loss and loss of appetite may be a knock-on effect of other side-effects. At a time when you need to conserve as much strength as you can, you may not feel like eating. You might try to eat small amounts more frequently than usual, and try to supplement your diet with high-calorie drinks to add extra calories.

Other side-effects vary, depending on the area of your body that is being treated, and your doctors will be able to provide you with information about the type of side-effects you might experience. For example, if you are having radiotherapy to the head or neck area you may suffer some hair loss. This is confined to the area being treated and the hair should grow back when your treatment has finished, but in some cases the hair loss may be permanent. It may also cause your mouth to become sore and more prone to infection than usual and the nurses caring for you will show you how to take extra care of your mouth during your treatment. Your sense of taste may also be affected, although this will gradually return to normal after your treatment ends. Radiotherapy to the abdominal region may cause some diarrhoea and inflammation of the bladder and cause you to feel a burning sensation when you pass urine. You may experience some nausea, and your appetite may be affected. Radiotherapy to the chest area may cause some tightness in your chest, which makes it more difficult than usual to swallow, but this should get better within a couple of months.

Effects on your life

The degree to which radiotherapy affects your daily life will depend very much upon the nature of your radiotherapy and how you respond to it. It is very important to remember that there is no 'right' way to live through this process, and that both the emotional and the physical effects will vary from person to person. Some people prefer to continue with as normal a routine as their radiotherapy schedule and physical energy will allow, as this helps them to retain some sense of control over their lives. For others, this may not be physically possible, or they may decide to make quite dramatic changes to their lives so that their time and energy is focused around their treatment. Most people will fall somewhere between the two. It will take time to adjust as the radiotherapy progresses, and you will need the support of family and friends. Don't be afraid to accept offers of help, either at home or driving you to your hospital appointments, for example.

Following surgery, Gary underwent an intensive course of radiotherapy for a tumour which had recurred in his brain. His treatment was given twice a day, morning and afternoon, as an out-patient on Monday to Friday over four weeks.

As I lived some distance from the hospital, I stayed with a friend for the duration of my treatment, going home only at weekends. The radiotherapy made me very tired and lethargic, and I had to make the journey to the hospital by public transport twice a day – I was not allowed to drive because of the possible effects of my tumour. Friends helped out by driving me to or from the hospital when they could, but it was hard to stay motivated and believe that the treatment would be worth all the effort. I didn't suffer too badly from other side-effects, although eating sensibly, keeping myself occupied (other than sleeping) and generally looking after myself were hard work. The point of relating this is not to put other people off, but to emphasize that sometimes you need more support and encouragement than you appreciate at the beginning of your treatment. You just have to keep remembering (and it helps if other people repeat it) that it is just too important not to see it through. Against the odds, I have been completely clear of cancer for over a year now.

Coping with your cancer and its treatment is discussed in more detail later in the book.

When your treatment has finished, your progress will be monitored via regular check-ups. It is extremely important for you to attend these appointments, as it is your main means of contact with your doctors. The knowledge that you will be attending check-ups on a long-term basis can be very reassuring. These appointments are a good opportunity to talk about any worries or queries which have arisen and you should never feel afraid to contact your doctor between appointments if you have a specific problem.

Chemotherapy

Chemotherapy might be proposed either as your sole form of treatment, or in combination with radiotherapy and/or surgery.

Chemotherapy literally means 'chemical therapy' and involves the use of cytotoxic (cell poisoning) drugs. There are many types of chemotherapy drugs, which, in broad terms, work by preventing cancer cells from growing and dividing, interfering with the reproduction process so that the cells become damaged and cannot reproduce themselves. The reason why there are so many different drugs is that they damage cancer cells in different ways. Different combinations of drugs have been shown to be effective in treating different cancers, and the drugs which you are given will be chosen on the basis of that research and experience.

The effectiveness of the drugs varies depending on your type of cancer and how advanced it is, and how sensitive the cancer cells prove to be to the chemotherapy drugs. This is difficult to predict until the chemotherapy is underway, and you will be carefully monitored throughout your treatment. In some cases, a complete cure may be possible and in others the aim may be to shrink the cancer as much as possible while not eliminating it completely. Your doctors will be best placed to advise you on the anticipated outcome for your particular treatment, although they will not be able to provide you with any guarantees.

Chemotherapy drugs can be given in different ways:

- by mouth in tablet form;
- by injection, into either the skin, the muscle or a vein. An intravenous drip into a vein is the most common route. This involves the insertion of a needle into a vein in your arm, and this

is attached to a fine tube through which the drugs flow. The drugs will often be diluted in liquid, and administered by a pump which carefully controls the rate at which you receive the drugs: this may be a few hours or up to a few days. The needle and tube are removed at the end of each treatment. In some cases, a tube is inserted into a vein in your chest (under anaesthetic, usually local), and this can be kept in place for the duration of your course of chemotherapy. This avoids the need for needles to be inserted in your arm for each treatment. You will be shown how to keep the line clean and to prevent it blocking between treatments;

- by infusion pump. This is similar to an intravenous drip, but involves using a portable pump which you can take home with you. It is small enough to be carried around with you in a bag or special belt, and allows controlled doses of drugs to be released into your bloodstream over a longer period – often 24 hours a day, seven days a week, for weeks at a time – without the need to stay in hospital for the duration of the treatment.

Depending on your chemotherapy regimen, you may have your drugs as an out-patient or you may need to stay in hospital for a few days. Chemotherapy is generally given as a number of cycles of treatment, each one lasting from between less than an hour to a few days. You will then have a rest period of up to a few weeks which allows the normal healthy tissue in your body to recover before your next treatment.

There is a general perception that undergoing chemotherapy is a particularly nasty experience, and that unpleasant side-effects such as prolonged nausea and vomiting cannot be avoided. It is worth remembering that not everybody suffers from all the side-effects of any given treatment, and that the medical staff will be trained and experienced in caring for patients having chemotherapy. They will do all they can to make you as comfortable as possible, and if you do suffer any problems, you should let them know as they may well be able to give you drugs to counteract your side-effects.

Side-effects

Many chemotherapy drugs damage not only the cancer cells but to a lesser extent other cells in the body which grow and reproduce rapidly, which is why you may suffer from side-effects from your treatment. The areas which tend to be affected are:

37

- digestive system, including the mouth. You may experience some nausea or sickness, although this depends on your drugs and can also vary from person to person. In any case, you will be offered anti-sickness drugs, which are extremely effective for many people in preventing sickness completely. It is important to stress that chemotherapy does not necessarily cause sickness, and that many patients nowadays have none at all. Your bowel habits may also be affected: diarrhoea and sometimes constipation can be caused by the effects of chemotherapy drugs. You may also find that your mouth becomes very tender, or that you develop mouth ulcers;
- bone marrow, which produces new red and white blood cells and platelets. You will have regular blood tests throughout your treatment to monitor your 'blood count'. If your red blood cell count is low, you may find that you become very tired, as the amount of oxygen being carried around your body is less than normal. This can be successfully treated by a blood transfusion. If your white cell count is low, you will be more prone to infection than usual, as the white cells are responsible for fighting off bacteria. This can be treated with antibiotics, if necessary. If your platelet count is low, you will find you bleed more than usual from minor cuts, and bruise more easily than normal. This can be treated by a platelet transfusion, which will help your blood to clot more easily;
- hair. Some – although not all – chemotherapy drugs cause hair loss, which many people find a very distressing prospect. This is probably the most widely known side-effect of chemotherapy because it is so visible. However, it is not the case that all chemotherapy drugs cause hair loss, and you should check with your doctor rather than assuming this will happen to you. Perhaps one of the reasons people find hair loss difficult to face is that it provides a constant reminder of your cancer, even if you are otherwise feeling relatively strong and well. Your hair will start to fall out a few weeks after your chemotherapy starts, and it will almost always grow back again once your treatment is completed.

There may also be more specific side-effects associated with your chemotherapy drugs: the staff who are nursing you will discuss these with you before your treatment starts.

Effects on your life

Different people react in different ways to their chemotherapy. Having to spend time in hospital either as an in-patient or an out-patient will inevitably lead to some disruption of your normal life. There may be times when you feel low physically or emotionally, and you will need extra support from family and friends. On the other hand, there may be times when you feel stronger and are able to work or follow your usual daily routine. The trick is to recognize when your body is at a low point (your doctors will be able to advise you about this), and not to try to fight it. You will recover more easily between cycles of treatment if you don't try to pretend that your body is at full strength. Do take it easy and rest when you need to: you will find that your body responds better if you take notice of what it is telling you. Of course, this is easier in theory than practice, and it is discussed in more detail in Chapter 7.

Neil underwent four separate courses of chemotherapy. The first was a 'standard' regimen for testicular cancer which lasted six cycles and initially appeared very successful. The others comprised different combinations of drugs to try to bring his cancer under control after it recurred.

I had no idea what to expect from chemotherapy, or even what it looked like. At first, I had a needle inserted in a vein in my arm, and the drugs were infused from a drip through a tube into the needle. Because of other complications, it was soon decided to insert a Hickman Line in my chest and my chemotherapy was administered through the line. The idea of a length of tube protruding from my chest was not a pleasant prospect, but it is surprising how quickly you get used to these things! When I went home, I was taught how to keep it free of blockages by 'flushing' it, and this simply became part of my routine. Not being allowed to soak in the bath was a minor source of irritation as the line has to be kept clear of germs, but this was not a big deal in the overall scheme of things.

I tolerated my first chemotherapy regimen relatively well and had few side-effects other than losing my hair – not a major issue for me in the context of getting rid of my cancer, although some people feel differently. The same applied to the second course. But the third was another story. I was very sick, which meant I didn't feel like eating for several days – although I was more than aware of the need to 'keep my strength up'. My recovery time between cycles was greater and maintaining levels of resolve and determination was, at times, an effort.

This period was hard work but I had learned by now not to fight the effects of these drugs. Our lives were pretty quiet for a while – coping with my cancer and treatment took a great deal of our time and energy. But we stuck together and managed, and made the most of my 'good' days. When my chemo 'cocktail' was changed again, most of my side-effects disappeared, and life became much more normal once more.

Other forms of treatment

Hormone therapy

Some cancers depend on a supply of hormones for their growth. The most common example of this in women is breast cancer and in men is prostate cancer, which needs testosterone in order to grow: without it, many tumours will shrink. Hormone therapy may therefore be recommended, which for prostate cancer takes the form of treatment either with hormones, or with drugs which interfere with the production or action of testosterone.

Hormone therapy is not used for the majority of cancers. As with all cancer treatments, any side-effects will depend upon the type of hormone therapy used, and if it is proposed for you, then your doctors will explain to you any side-effects which you might expect.

Biological therapy

There are hopes that various forms of biological therapy – and particularly those which help to stimulate the body's own immune system – may produce effective new treatments in the future, but research is still at a relatively early stage in most cases. It is hoped that in the future, treatments based on substances produced by the body – such as certain antibodies and interferons (substances produced by the immune system which have the ability to inhibit viral growth) – may be developed to supplement and complement existing treatments. For example, research continues to work on 'magic bullet' techniques, in which certain antibodies (known as monoclonal antibodies) carry cell-poisoning drugs or radioactive isotopes directly to cancer cells while leaving normal cells alone.

Alternative and complementary therapies

Forms of so-called 'alternative' therapy such as herbal, vitamin and dietary treatments, acupuncture and the use of homeopathic remedies are not yet proven as cancer treatments as they have not yet proven beneficial in the same lengthy and rigorous testing and trial processes as conventional cancer treatments. However, all doctors know that some drugs used today are based on traditional remedies or plant extracts – including some heart drugs and some anti-cancer drugs. A good doctor will be open-minded and, once tests prove an 'alternative' remedy to be effective, there is no reason why it should not enter 'mainstream' medicine.

Even before that, some alternative therapies may hold considerable attraction given the nature of conventional cancer treatments, and there are increasing numbers of practitioners of non-conventional medicine. Some people find that they do derive some benefit from undergoing alternative therapies, and claims have been made for the effectiveness of, for example, certain homeopathic remedies in boosting the strength of the immune system. There is as yet no concrete evidence (as recognized by the conventional medical profession) that any alternative therapy will contribute to the success of a conventional cancer treatment, but if it contributes to your overall well-being, then there may be a strong motivation to consider it. It is very important to consult your oncologist before embarking on any complementary treatment, and to appreciate that alternative therapies do not aim to replicate the effects of conventional treatments.

On another level, you may find therapies such as massage, aromatherapy and relaxation techniques (which do not claim any specific healing properties) may still be beneficial to your overall well-being. Massage of areas of tension such as the shoulders can promote physical and mental relaxation. Learning breathing or visualization techniques which help your mind to slow down and let go of your worries for a short time can also be helpful. You may well find that classes are organized by your hospital, or that staff can provide you with information about useful contacts. Again, it is wise to check with your doctor before undergoing any physical therapies, in case they aggravate certain physical symptoms.

'Prevention is better than cure'

Most of us are well aware of preventive measures which can help to reduce the risk of developing certain cancers. If you, as a reader, are already living with cancer then you might feel 'This doesn't apply to me – I've already got cancer' and feel disinclined to be lectured about your lifestyle and behaviour, past or present. This is not a lecture, nor does it assume a right to tell people how to live their lives. It is simply a reminder that some of the main contributing 'behavioural' factors to certain types of cancer are smoking, excessive exposure to sunlight, alcohol and a low-fibre, high-fat diet. It is also unwise to dismiss the relevance of attendance at screening programmes, if appropriate.

4

Dealing with your medical team

Depending on the type and stage of your cancer, your diagnosis may have been made very quickly following a referral by your GP to your local hospital, or you may have undergone a series of tests lasting some weeks before a firm diagnosis is reached. In both cases, you will have been through an extremely stressful experience and have been thrust into a medical world with which you are likely to be completely unfamiliar.

Studies have shown that men are less likely than women to visit their GP when they fall ill. As a result, you may have had infrequent contact with doctors in the past, and be unaccustomed to discussing and managing ill-health and dealing with the medical profession. In spite of this, you not only have to cope with the news of your cancer diagnosis, but also learn about your disease, learn your way around the unfamiliar territory of hospitals and clinics, learn how to talk to unfamiliar doctors about even the most intimate and distressing aspects of your illness, learn about your proposed treatment, learn a new vocabulary of medical terms and jargon . . . It would be a lot to ask of any person in normal circumstances, and yet it is a process which you have to come to terms with in a very short time.

This sounds extremely daunting and the learning curve is a steep one, but there are simple ways in which you can begin to feel more involved in the management of your cancer rather than falling prey to the passivity which many male (and female) patients fear. The key to this is communication with your medical team.

Who's who

It may feel at times that a whole range of doctors, nurses and other specialists are involved in your treatment, making it hard to establish a constructive 'working' relationship with any of them. At first it can be difficult enough just to learn their names and what their role is. Once your diagnosis has been made and your treatment begins, this problem should ease as you become more familiar with the staff on your ward or at your clinic if you are being treated as an out-patient.

In most hospitals, you will be assigned a consultant who is in charge of your care, and who may be one of several attached to your ward or clinic. Indeed, you may see more than one consultant if you are undergoing surgery as part of your treatment: you may have an oncology consultant responsible for your overall treatment, with a different specialist consultant in charge of your operation. Working for the consultants are a number of registrars who are doctors at various levels of seniority, and more junior doctors known as house officers. If yours is a teaching hospital, student doctors may also observe your care from time to time.

If you are undergoing radiotherapy, you will have contact with the specialist staff in that department who will administer your treatment each day. Men undergoing chemotherapy will be looked after during their treatment by specially trained oncology nurses, who are skilled both in administering chemotherapy drugs and looking after people affected by cancer. If you are treated as an in-patient, oncology nurses play a vital role in your day-to-day care.

You may also spend time at the X-ray department having scans or X-rays; a dietician can help if you have difficulties eating or with your diet; social workers are attached to the hospital to help sort out financial difficulties or benefits; physiotherapists can provide support with issues related to mobility and maintaining physical activity; occupational therapists can help and advise with special equipment or changes to your home which will make your daily life more comfortable; counsellors will be available to offer support. These are just some of the specialist services available to you as a patient, and which you can draw upon at any time. You may or may not need their expertise, but it is reassuring to know that they exist.

Outside the hospital, your GP will be kept informed of your treatment, and a district nurse will be available to visit you at home if needed and provide additional support. Depending on your circumstances and how unwell you are, Macmillan nurses or Marie Curie nurses can offer information, general support and specialist care at home if you need it.

While this may seem an excessively long list of people to be involved in the care of a single patient, it is also an indication of the sheer breadth of resources available to help and support you. While you may have contact with only a few of them throughout most of your treatment, it is important to know that your hospital can provide support with a variety of cancer-related issues, from pain-relief to dietary advice to financial advice. Do use these specialist skills when you need them!

The early stages

Most people are referred by their GP to their local hospital to carry out the first stages of investigation and diagnosis. You will probably be given the results of your tests by the specialist who examined you at the hospital. Even if you had suspected that your health problem was serious, a diagnosis of cancer still comes as a tremendous shock, and you will need time to absorb the medical details which are related to you. Everybody's experience is different so Neil's is not necessarily typical, although the sense of shock is shared by most.

I am afraid that there is really no way around that dreadful moment when the C-word is first used, and I am not convinced that there is a 'best' way in which it can be handled. I had been urgently referred to our nearest Accident & Emergency unit, but neither my partner nor I really had any idea why we were driving some 15 miles to hospital, having no inkling of the nature of the problem or its implications. We spent hours waiting in a side room while the house officer on duty tried to find time to diagnose me between more urgent calls.

Much later, it happened. A surgeon came in to examine me, felt my abdomen and testicles and announced without preamble, 'I think it's testicular cancer.' He looked at our shocked faces and informed us, 'Well, you wouldn't have wanted it told to you any other way, would you?' Like the first moment when a wave knocks you off your feet as a toddler at the seaside and you swallow a mouthful of seawater and struggle in panic to breathe again, this is a defining moment. The only question I could think of asking was 'How long?'

'With treatment, maybe a year or two. Without treatment, about six months.' And that was that. Diagnosis complete. Neither of us had a clue how to face this.

The next few hours passed in a blur of X-rays and ultrasound scans which confirmed the surgeon's diagnosis. We then left the hospital, with appointments for a CT scan the following afternoon and an operation to remove the testicle and primary tumour a few days later, but without the painkillers I had been promised.

It was several weeks later that a different consultant at a different hospital gave us the relatively joyous news that he put my chances of a complete recovery at about 50:50. This was a different picture altogether, and gave us something more tangible to hold onto and fight for now.

However sensitively and carefully you are told the news about your cancer, you will probably be aware only of an immense, almost physical sense of shock. How much information you subsequently take in during your consultation is bound to be limited, but even at this stage it is important to try to understand what your doctors tell you. This may sound harsh as it can be difficult to interpret what doctors are saying, even if they are clear in their information from a medical point of view. For example, if you are told that an X-ray or scan shows a shadow or lesions, or that a blood test shows abnormal levels of proteins or hormones or that you are anaemic, this may not necessarily mean much to you as a lay-person, and especially in terms of your cancer diagnosis. You are unlikely to feel like taking charge of the consultation and asking probing questions in scientific terms. Most of us do not have the medical background to be able to do so, and in these circumstances you may well not be capable of your usual rational thought processes.

Becoming accustomed to medical jargon is one hurdle to be crossed. You can't be expected to be familiar with much of the terminology you hear, and it can feel as if you are being blinded with science. Asking for terms to be explained is essential because those same terms are likely to arise again and again. Bear in mind too that while you may feel frustrated at your need to say – yet again – 'Could you just explain exactly what that means, please?', doctors need to be precise and accurate in the information they give you and hence need to draw on the appropriate precise and accurate medical terms. It would be even more frustrating simply to be told, 'There's something a bit odd going on in your stomach/chest/blood.' A glossary of the terms you are most likely to encounter is included at the end of the book.

Although it can feel like hard work, do try to make sure you have a basic understanding of what you have been told, so that you are not left wondering later if you have remembered correctly. If you attend the consultation alone, you might even try to make a few written notes of the main points and check with your doctor that these are accurate. This approach does not suit everybody, but is a useful habit if you can manage it. If you have a member of your family or a close friend with you and you are happy for them to sit in on your consultation, then they can help by playing a 'listening' role for you or by taking notes. At some hospitals it is possible to make a tape recording of your out-patient consultations with doctors which you can play back later.

The process of communication at this early stage is critical, and has to work both ways: not only do you need to understand what you are told, but you need to be able to describe to your doctor how you are feeling. This might include both general and specific points such as:

- how you feel generally – basically well, or run down, or suffering weight loss, etc;
- your specific physical symptoms – cough, headache, digestive problems, difficulties with mobility, lumps in or on the skin, etc;
- whether you have any pain, where it is and what type it is (occasional, constant, stabbing, dull, etc).

If you have previously visited your doctor's surgery only rarely, it can be difficult to find the right words to describe how you are feeling and it can be tempting to leave out information because it seems trivial or because you feel embarrassed. It can be equally tempting to overstate your symptoms or problems to ensure that they are not overlooked, but this is more likely to cause confusion – if you have an occasional pain, try not to give the impression that it is continuous and unbearable! Don't worry that you can't use medical terms: it is more important that you are clear, accurate and as factual as possible in your account and that your doctor has an adequate picture of your problems.

Doctors should always ask you if you have any questions, and at this early stage it can be difficult to formulate exactly what you want to know, when you are still feeling the effects of the initial shock. If you do have specific concerns – especially if you are experiencing any pain – then it is important that these are addressed, and that you feel that you are being listened to. Going home without asking the one key question which has been bothering you for a fortnight will only cause you additional stress in the days to come. You certainly should not feel that the doctors are too busy to spend time answering your questions. They have many demands on their time, but they do want to offer you the maximum possible help and they cannot do this to the full if you feel afraid to discuss your concerns and queries with them.

You may be offered information in the form of leaflets to read at your leisure or the opportunity to talk to a specially trained nurse about your cancer. Your GP will also be kept informed about your diagnosis, and may be able to offer support or details of organizations which can provide you with more detailed information about your cancer. If you are not offered any help of this type and you feel it would benefit you, then do ask. All hospitals should at the very least be able to help you to find written information even if they cannot provide it themselves.

You may well need further tests before your treatment can begin, and the timescale will depend on your hospital and the nature of your cancer. In some cases, a delay of several weeks may be of little consequence and in others it will be necessary to act more quickly. The doctors looking after you should ensure that you receive your care at an appropriate time, but if you feel that delays are occurring for no good reason, then do not be afraid to mention this. You may find that there is a valid reason why tests are not scheduled immediately or your next consultation will not take place for a fortnight. Perhaps test samples have to be sent away to another lab for investigation, for example.

Time can easily become a big issue, especially in retrospect. From a doctor's viewpoint, apparent delays are likely to stem from one of two reasons. First, there is a medical need to be sure that the diagnosis is correct. One oncologist commented that most doctors can think of little worse from a patient's point of view than being told erroneously, 'You have cancer' and then, later, 'No, it's all right. Just a mistake. You don't.' Secondly, even after the initial diagnosis has been made, it is still incomplete from a medical viewpoint. For example, different types and extents of cancer need different treatments (there are several types of lung cancer, bladder cancer and testicular cancer, to name just a few), and further tests may therefore be necessary to define the exact type or extent. If you understand these reasons, you will have one less worry in the meantime. With the benefit of hindsight, Neil felt he might have avoided a very distressing week by asking more questions.

After the surgical removal of my testicle, there was a terrible period of 12 days before I was admitted to a specialist cancer unit as an emergency. In retrospect, we did not make anywhere near enough noise to try to force the issue during that time. But we were still deeply in shock, trying to find out more about this cancer and desperately trying to keep on top of the practical details of our lives. While it was quite obvious to me that I was deteriorating rapidly, we assumed that the medical profession knew best, and if they said 'Wait at home', then we would wait at home. Although we were trying to be sensible and co-operative, to the extent of making written notes about my particular problems, when we did have a hospital consultation the week after my operation nobody wanted to listen to us. The details of my diagnosis (whether my testicular cancer was of the seminoma or teratoma type) were not yet available, and therefore I did not appear to exist as a cancer patient.

A further week later, I attended a cancer clinic at the hospital. The details of my diagnosis were confirmed, and at last a cancer specialist was listening to me. I was in constant pain and could no longer eat at all. She examined me briefly, arranged for X-rays to be taken and arranged for me to be admitted to the cancer unit of a hospital some 30 miles away, as an emergency patient.

The point of relating this experience is not to heap criticism on the medical profession – although a little more support would have made a huge difference. What is more important is to know when to make a fuss, and not to be afraid to do it. Consultations can be brought forward, stronger pain-killers can be provided – it is *not* asking too much. Unfortunately, you may only develop the confidence to stand up and make your views known much later.

It is likely that you will see more than one doctor during the testing and diagnostic process. You may feel that you undergo the same physical examination and description of your symptoms and history over and over again. This can feel frustrating, and it helps if you understand the role of the various different doctors in your care. For example, you may see a specialist in treating the part of the body in question (such as a urologist or a chest specialist) and also an oncologist (a cancer specialist). Indeed, you may see several doctors at different levels of seniority from each of these departments, and it can take some time to work out where they fit into the hospital hierarchy. They should always introduce themselves to you, but again, do not be afraid to ask them about their role in your care: they may be involved only in your diagnosis, for example, or in a longer term role in the treatment of your cancer. They may be instrumental in reaching decisions about your diagnosis and treatment, or they may have a more junior role.

One vitally important issue your doctors should address early on is the potential need for sperm collection and banking. If they do not, then you should not feel shy to bring up the subject yourself: it is too important an issue to be passed over. Some chemotherapy drugs and radiotherapy treatments can affect your fertility and if you have not yet had children or feel that you may wish to have more children in the future, then you may need to consider sperm banking. This should be discussed with you at an early stage if it is appropriate: once treatment is underway, then it may be too late. In some cases, fertility may gradually return after treatment is completed, but sperm banking will act as an insurance policy if this is not the case. This is a difficult and emotive issue, particularly for relatively young men who had assumed that they would one day father children without the need for medical intervention, and you may find it difficult to discuss with relative strangers. It may also be that you already feel saturated with bad news and would rather not face yet another problematic issue. Do try to talk about it, not just with your doctors but also with your spouse or partner and remember that it may be an extremely valuable insurance policy in years to come.

Developing relationships with medical practitioners

It may take some time before you feel sufficiently at ease in a hospital environment to take full advantage of the knowledge and expertise of the medical team treating you. A sense that events are completely beyond your control – and knowledge – is a common reaction, and it is easy to become very passive as a patient. For many men, this is an alien sensation and all the more difficult to deal with as a result. Most of us are accustomed to a regular routine in which we are largely in control of most aspects of our life, be it in a job or home life. It can be particularly disturbing to find that your life has been turned upside down by your cancer diagnosis, and that you have lost the security of your 'normal' life, even if it had its own problems and sources of stress.

Developing the desire and the confidence to talk to doctors will take time, especially if, like many people, you feel slightly in awe of them or not sufficiently comfortable to talk naturally to them. First you have to want to talk and to ask questions. Then you have to get used to having conversations which do not necessarily tell you what you want to hear. If there is one doctor who you find more sympathetic and easier to talk to than the others involved in your treatment, you might start by talking to him or her. You may also need to work out (or ask!) which staff are most involved with your treatment and care and are therefore likely to be best informed about your particular situation.

As in any other aspect of life or work, some medical practitioners are easier to talk to than others. Do not be put off if a doctor does not appear particularly forthcoming and communicative: it may be that they are trying to judge just how much information you would like to be given or are able to absorb rather than simply bombarding you with medical jargon. The medical terms they use are likely to be unfamiliar at first, and it may be some time before you are fully conversant with them. Don't be afraid to ask for more explanation, or for information to be repeated if you have not fully understood the first time. A glossary of some of the terms you may encounter is included at the end of the book.

Inevitably, you will think of important questions between consultations or hospital visits and it is very easy to forget them when you are face to face with your doctor. You will, of course, remember them as soon as your meeting is over! To avoid this problem, you may find it helpful to make a written note of your questions, and also of any problems which you experience between hospital visits or treatments. For example, if you are experiencing new or different pain, then your doctors may be able to prescribe alternative medication to combat this. (Obviously, if you are suffering serious pain then you should contact your doctor or hospital straight away.) Similarly, if you are having difficulty maintaining a reasonable diet or eating sufficient in quantity, it is important to let your doctor know as hospital dieticians may be able to offer you advice about boosting your diet. Some people find that a small notebook is easier than scraps of paper (which can easily get lost) for writing down short notes to use as an *aide-mémoire*.

After my initial diagnosis, we never attended another consultation or meeting without a notebook and a list of questions. Helen, my partner, carried this notebook with her everywhere and Volume One soon filled with the details of test results, planned treatment, progress of treatment, changes in treatment – in fact, all the factual information passed on to us. We wrote down queries between hospital visits or as they occurred to us while I was in hospital, and often ran through our 'agenda' in the car on our way to consultations. In this sense, I suppose we treated them as we would a business meeting. It was also a tremendous help when we were discussing progress together or with, for example, my parents, because we always had something concrete to refer to.

Talking to doctors

In the early stages, you may feel that you simply don't know what questions to ask about your cancer and treatment, beyond a general sense of 'What's going to happen to me?' When your doctors ask you, 'Do you have any questions?' it can be difficult to know where to begin, and how to put your fears and queries into words without appearing foolish or stupid. Most people are starting from a base of no knowledge at all on the subject of their cancer, so it may be most constructive to begin with some very basic questions, which you can develop as your knowledge builds up. For example:

- How do your doctors know that you have cancer?
- What type of cancer do you have and how advanced is it?
- How does it spread and how will it affect your body and the functioning of your organs?
- What type of treatment is proposed?
- How long is the treatment likely to take? (weeks? months?)
- What is the hoped-for outcome of the treatment (although it is never possible for doctors to give guarantees)? Is a cure or substantial remission a possibility or is the treatment palliative (aiming to alleviate but not to cure)?
- How will the progress of your treatment be measured?
- Who is the doctor who will be in charge of your treatment? Are there any other doctors you will see on a regular basis?
- Where will you receive your treatment? Will you have to stay in hospital?

Asking a few specific questions such as these will often help to prompt further information from your doctor. It is easy otherwise for a consultation to speed by before you feel sufficiently at ease to really start talking. Remember that you don't have to talk in medical jargon, although you do need to be clear. It's perfectly acceptable to say, 'I have a sharp pain in my stomach' – you are not expected to be able to perform self-diagnosis. On the other hand, it is helpful if you know the names and doses of any drugs you are taking (for pain relief, anti-nausea, etc), so that your doctor can check on their effectiveness and whether any prescriptions need to be changed. This is less daunting than it sounds, as you will be given a card containing details of your drugs, which should be kept up to date. It is much easier if you can discuss these by name rather than 'the big pink capsules' or 'the little yellow pills'.

The question many people consider the most important – and the most difficult to ask – is on the subject of your future prognosis. In the past, a cancer diagnosis was an almost certain death sentence, and many people still make this association immediately on hearing their diagnosis. However, treatments have progressed tremendously in recent years, and it may be that your cancer can be treated effectively. This depends, of course, on your type of cancer, how advanced it is and how you as an individual respond to treatment. When you ask about your likely prognosis, your doctor may use terms whose meaning is not obvious to you, but which have a specific connotation in this context. These include 'cure', 'remission' and 'relapse'.

• *Cure*

A cure means that all evidence of your cancer has been eliminated completely and that it will not return. How this is assessed depends on the type of cancer in question. For example, testicular cancer tends to recur within five years, and most often within two or three. So if your initial treatment is successful and a period of five years passes in which no cancer is detected, you should be considered cured. Other cancers recur in different timescales, and your doctor will be able to advise you about this.

• *Remission*

Remission means that the symptoms of your cancer have disappeared or lessened, i.e. that the cancer has got smaller. A partial remission means that the cancer has shrunk by at least half. A complete remission means that the evidence of your cancer has disappeared completely and it is no longer detectable. This is not the same as a cure, as the cancer may return in the future. If it does not return within a given timespan, you may be considered cured.

• *Relapse/Recurrence*

This means that following your treatment, some cancer cells still remained in your body and started to grow into a detectable cancer again. It may be that these remaining cancer cells were undetectable after your initial treatment but have become active again later. This can occur in the months after treatment has ended or may not happen for some years. Your doctors will advise you about the likelihood of a relapse occurring.

You might be eager to know about your chances of achieving a cure or substantial remission, but this may be tempered by a fear of hearing bad news – for example, that only a short period of remission is expected to be achieved by treatment. Your doctors may volunteer information about the anticipated success of your treatment, based both on statistical information and the specific details of your own case.

Another term you will hear doctors refer to is the 'stage' of your cancer, which describes the extent, if any, to which it has spread to other parts of your body. There are four stages. Stage I means there is no spread and the cancer is confined to the primary site. Stage IV means that there is extensive spread beyond the primary site. Stages II and III fall between the two extremes.

Some people want to be kept fully informed about the progress of their treatment. You may decide, on the other hand, that you do not wish to be told too much medical detail about your cancer and treatment, especially at first. This is a very personal choice and is entirely your decision. Your doctors should be sensitive to this, although they do need to ensure that you understand what is happening during your treatment and afterwards.

It is worth remembering that while you will be looking for definitive answers to your questions, it may sometimes be difficult for your doctors to provide them. This does not mean that they are avoiding your questions, or that there are gaps in their knowledge. The treatment of cancer holds many uncertainties, and it would be wrong for doctors to be asked to provide guarantees about the future, although it is natural for you – and your family – to seek reassurance. It is useful to find out at an early stage which doctors you will have greatest contact with, so that you know who is likely to have the most knowledge about your case and is therefore in the best position to answer your questions.

In the very early stages, you may feel that you want to know as little about your cancer and treatment as possible and that additional information and knowledge are pointless because they can make no difference to your condition. This is a perfectly understandable reaction as you and your family try to come to terms with your diagnosis. As the initial shock recedes, however, you are likely to find that it is helpful to start learning a little more about your cancer. There are many books and leaflets available, covering a huge range of cancer-related topics. For some basic factual information, your hospital should be able to provide you with booklets produced by the organization BACUP (British Association of Cancer United Patients). These cover both specific cancers and related issues, such as cancer treatments and diet. Books and leaflets have a useful role as you can refer to them when you please.

If you are unclear about information you have received, you should never be afraid to ask your medical team for clarification. Similarly, don't worry about asking the same questions more than once: when you are under stress, it is sometimes difficult to absorb information as easily as usual and your medical team will understand this.

Dealing with pain

One of the main fears of many cancer patients is that they will suffer prolonged and uncontrollable pain. This should not be the case as advances both in understanding of the causes of pain and in methods of pain relief mean that pain can be effectively treated in most cases.

The nature of our society is such that men are encouraged to be physically strong and to shrug off pain, so the acknowledgement of a fear of pain or actual pain is not necessarily an easy matter. Most of us can tolerate some degree of pain for a short time: the pain from toothache or sporting injuries is unpleasant but we generally know that it will be short-lived. Pain resulting from a serious illness is a different matter, partly because of its physical effects and also because of the fear which arises from the inability to control what is happening within your own body. Around a third of people who have cancer suffer no pain at all. For those who do experience some pain, it can generally be controlled extremely effectively.

There are some people for whom a fear of needles (needle phobia) is a source of discouragement from admitting to pain, as they are very much afraid of being subjected to painkilling injections. This is a perfectly valid fear, and one which should be treated sympathetically by medical staff. Furthermore, there are many forms of pain relief which do not require any injections so you should not be afraid to voice your fear to your medical team. In fact, many people manage to overcome their fear.

The degree of pain or discomfort you experience is not necessarily an indicator of how advanced your cancer is. Pain is often not caused by a tumour per se but because, for example, the tumour is pressing on its surrounding tissues or on a nerve. The pain caused by pressure on a nerve may manifest itself in a part of the body quite remote from the tumour site. Pain may also be caused by other factors, such as

• infection;
• because a tumour is obstructing the normal action of your bowel;
• because of a secondary tumour in a bone.

We all have different levels of pain tolerance, and in any case, people with the same type of cancer may not have the same symptoms or experience of pain or discomfort. For this reason, it is very important for you to be able to describe your particular pain to your medical team so that they can treat it in the most effective way possible. As with your other symptoms, it is easy to overstate or understate pain depending on your frame of mind that day, so keeping a written note of the points you want to tell your doctors may help.

Describing pain is not easy especially if it is quite severe and you just want a doctor to make it disappear. There are a number of points that will be helpful to doctors in working out what is causing your pain and therefore in prescribing the most effective form of pain relief:

• Where do you feel the pain? Does it spread?

- What type of pain is it – a continuous dull ache, a brief stabbing pain or a burning sensation, for example?
- Do you have the pain all the time or does it come and go? How long does it last? Does it keep you awake or can you sleep through it?
- Does anything make the pain worse – eating or drinking, moving around, coughing, lifting or stretching?
- Does anything make the pain better – painkillers (what sort?), lying down, keeping still, heat or cold?

Analysing your own pain in terms which help your doctors can be difficult and frustrating at first, especially when you are getting used to communicating with them – there may be times when you just want to shout at them to make it go away. Be assured that they genuinely want to ease your pain, and will do all they can to do so.

Painkilling drugs

Painkilling drugs – which are known as analgesics – are split into three categories: mild, moderate and strong. The mild medications include aspirin and paracetamol which can be very effective. The moderate analgesics are stronger and often work on the brain and nervous system, and include, for example, codeine-based medications. The most common painkillers in the strong group of analgesics are morphine and diamorphine. Many patients become fearful on two counts when they hear these names: they fear addiction and associate their use with the final stages of illness and the end of life. In these circumstances morphine is not addictive. If the cause of the pain is subsequently treated in some other way – for example, chemotherapy or radiotherapy reduces the tumour and relieves the pressure which caused the pain – then the morphine can be reduced or phased out. You will not be left with an addiction to the drug. Secondly, morphine is commonly used at a relatively early stage: its use is dependent on the level of pain a patient is suffering, and not on how advanced their cancer is. Incidentally, morphine is also used for pain caused by injuries and conditions other than cancer.

Painkillers may be used in combination with other drugs such as steroids, antibiotics or anti-depressants. While you may feel at times that you are taking more drugs than you would normally be comfortable with, it is more important to realize that each drug has a purpose, and that your 'cocktail' of medications will be tailored to your specific needs.

You may find that other methods are effective in conjunction with your medication in controlling your pain, and these can be physical or psychological. Physical alternatives might include:

- acupuncture;
- transcutaneous electrical nerve stimulation (TENS) which works by stimulating the nerves to release the body's natural pain-killers;
- gentle massage;
- nerve blocks.

Simply ensuring that you are physically comfortable can make a difference too. Check that your bed or chair gives you adequate support, that your posture is not contributing to your discomfort, that you are not too hot or too cold.

Your pain may be aggravated by tension and anxiety, and psychological methods can make a difference to your overall sense of well-being, and thus help to ease physical pain. Learning relaxation techniques can help you to feel less tense, and simply having someone to talk to openly can relieve stress, whether they are a professional counsellor or a friend. Time can weigh heavy too, and this can make you even more aware of pain or discomfort. You may find that the distraction of the television or radio, a good book or magazine, or a good friend to talk to can divert your mind, even if only for a short time.

Physical pain is unpleasant in any circumstances, but at a time when you are feeling particularly vulnerable, it can become a source of rage and distress as well. If you have always been reasonably fit and well, physical weakness is very frustrating and you may feel angry with yourself that you are not strong enough to disregard your pain and continue with your normal life. Having your family and friends see you in pain can feel humiliating, especially if you are accustomed to being a 'strong' person. You may feel similarly about needing to ask for help to accomplish small tasks because your pain prevents you from doing things yourself. It is not easy!

In the vast majority of cases, physical pain can be controlled effectively. It may be difficult to admit to your pain, but denying it or trying to manage without pain relief won't help you either to recover or to feel better. There is nothing to be gained by being 'brave'. You need all your energies to cope with your cancer and there is nothing to be gained by wasting valuable strength and energy in fighting pain.

5

Coping in the early stages

The hours and days immediately after your cancer diagnosis has been confirmed are in some ways the most difficult because it is now that your world is turned upside-down. This is the point at which the transition into new and frightening territory begins and the time when the sense of shock is at its most raw. You may already have experienced the considerable stress of tests to establish whether or not you have cancer and the sense of being in limbo as you await the results. Receiving a cancer diagnosis, however sensitively the news is given to you, represents the confirmation of your worst fears. You may be unwell and in pain or you may be physically able to continue your normal life. In either case, the period between diagnosis and the beginning of treatment can be a time of great upheaval, both practically and emotionally. Everybody reacts differently, but gradually you will need to find your own way of coming to terms with your cancer and working out how to live with it.

In the early days, the overwhelming emotion experienced by many people is shock. It can leave you feeling numb and dazed and can make absorbing information or taking decisions difficult. Some people start to feel that dealing with anything practical is completely superfluous, and just want someone to magic away their cancer and return their life to normal. Others are galvanized into action, and want to sort out the aspects of their life which will be affected by their cancer and treatment, such as their job or other regular commitments. Shock affects everybody differently, and there is no 'right' way to react to your cancer diagnosis. It will take time to accept it and the changes it will bring to your life, and this process cannot be rushed.

Neil's diagnosis had been made during the course of a single day, and he made an immediate and conscious decision not to allow this momentous event to impose on him the passivity which is often associated with being a hospital patient.

So that was it then. I was now back at home in a physical state which was exactly the same as when I left home to visit the hospital some eight hours earlier. There was the knowledge however that I had cancer and we had better start thinking about getting a few things sorted out. I think that this is probably the moment at which it is easiest for the patient either to empower themselves by becoming totally involved in the ghastly process or to abdicate responsibility by letting events run away from you. The decision is very often in the hands of the patient and his family and friends. Do not underestimate the importance of this point!

You may feel very alone and isolated after being told you have cancer. Your doctor or GP may try to reassure you with anecdotes about the effectiveness of treatment for your type of cancer or about other patients' experiences, but these can seem completely irrelevant to your particular situation. You might feel like the only person in the world who has ever been in such terrible circumstances. Some hospitals provide support for patients immediately after their diagnosis, such as a Macmillan nurse (who will be specially trained in helping cancer patients) or specialist counselling. You might think that talking further about your cancer cannot possibly help. After all, talking makes no difference to your diagnosis. In fact, talking to a medical professional other than the doctor who made your diagnosis can help you to start voicing your questions and fears: this in itself is a hurdle to be crossed. If the hospital has no such support system, then your GP should be happy to talk to you at short notice.

For some men, beginning to talk about a cancer diagnosis is not so easy in practice. If you are not in the habit of discussing such personal and private matters, your instinct may be that your cancer is nobody's business but yours. A temptation to feel that you must be strong and 'pull yourself together' is prevalent in many men, together with a sense that the need to seek outside help is a sign of weakness. These may be entirely unconscious reactions, born of habit, and it would be unreasonable to expect any man newly diagnosed with cancer to develop new ways of coping overnight. What is important is for both men and those close to them to be aware of the support available at this stage (it may not be widely publicized), and not to feel reticent about drawing on it whenever it is needed.

After your diagnosis has been made, simply leaving the hospital and getting through the rest of the day can feel impossibly difficult. What are you to do now? It can feel as if your entire world has just collapsed around you. You know that somehow you have to go home or back to work, and that the world around you is exactly as it was before your diagnosis – but for you it has changed irrevocably.

How you react at this time will be driven less by conscious decision than by instinct and the effects of shock. Returning to your normal routine might deflect the impact of your diagnosis for a short time. It is as if the action of going back to work or to the supermarket can push your diagnosis into the background for a while. You might need to spend some time alone to absorb the news and to think quietly about it before telling anybody. If your wife or partner or a close member of your family was with you when you heard your diagnosis, you might spend time alone with them, until you feel able to start passing on the news to others. Neil found he needed time for the news to sink in, but then some issues started to become clearer:

> There is a moment which seems to go on for ever on the first evening of 'C-Day' which is me and my partner sitting on our sofa just holding hands in absolute silence with nothing that we could possibly say. I do remember that it was that evening that we made what I am certain was the most important decision of this whole 'voyage': to take control in whatever ways we could. The need to attempt to regain some control over these events was the secondary emotional reaction after the trauma of the diagnosis.

The need for some sense of control is not uncommon, born of a fear that if you do not actively take control of what events you can, then events will surely take control of you. It is certainly not the only common reaction though; withdrawal into oneself can be hard to avoid too, especially if you are inclined not to talk openly about your feelings. 'I really don't want to talk about it' may be your overriding feeling, through a combination of shock and the difficulty of seeing a way forward through the treatment and uncertainty ahead.

Getting through the day is tough. Around you, all is normal – but your world has changed. You may be capable of little but sitting at home thinking through your consultation and diagnosis. You might need to use 'normal' activities to prevent yourself going over the same ground again and again in your mind, taking refuge in seemingly trivial tasks – walking the dog, cutting the grass, cleaning the car. This may seem odd behaviour to an onlooker, but can feel like the only way to cope with the immediate effects of shock as you try to come to terms with your diagnosis.

It is extremely important to find and use some support at this stage and especially so if you are alone. You may feel that you can cope on your own and neither need nor want to talk to anybody. Maybe you can manage, but you are likely to cope more effectively if you feel able to ask for support, and particularly someone to talk to at this early stage. Sitting at home on your own, worrying about your cancer and treatment and the future is a natural reaction, but ultimately it will not benefit you either physically or emotionally. You need to conserve all your strength to fight your disease and deal with your treatment, so now is not the moment to assert that you don't need any help from anybody. Even if you don't feel like talking, just the presence of a good friend or close family member can help to dissipate the sense that you are the only person in the world facing this problem.

Even if your thoughts are not very clear at this time, talking will help you more than bottling up your questions and fears. It may take some time before you can start to think clearly. You might find your thoughts go around in circles, stuck in a loop in which you can't get your diagnosis out of your mind, and simply don't know what to do with yourself. Perhaps you can't stop thinking 'Why me? What have I done to deserve this?', and want nothing more than for life to go back to normal, as it was yesterday or last week or last month. Talking will help to provide a release.

It is not always easy to find the right person to talk to, and you might feel awkward at first discussing your situation with those closest to you. Some people prefer to talk to a professional counsellor or a nurse or doctor about their disease in the first instance. If you are not offered counselling, your GP or your hospital should be able to help with this – and should also be able to advise you about other forms of practical and emotional support available to you.

Breaking the news

It is tempting to put off telling other people about your cancer because the task of breaking the bad news simply feels too much. You may also feel that if you tell no one, then your cancer feels less real – if you don't acknowledge it to the outside world, then somehow it doesn't exist. After coping with your diagnosis and trying to absorb the news yourself, finding the right words to tell other people is not easy. Men can be less forthcoming than women in talking about their health and less accustomed to sharing and discussing such personal details with family, friends or the medical profession. Whether or not your family and friends were aware that you had a health problem, you know that they will be deeply shocked and upset by your cancer diagnosis and this makes the news harder to break.

You may also feel a sense of guilt at causing them so much worry about such a serious health issue, and that you are responsible for inflicting this pain upon them. Perhaps you also feel guilty that your cancer is in some way your fault, that you have 'allowed' it to happen and you fear that people will blame you for it. This may be irrational, but when you are under such stress your thoughts and emotions will be very confused. However, putting off telling people is more likely to make these problems worse than better for you, and people who thought they were close to you may feel hurt and upset that you didn't feel able to talk to them sooner.

Who to tell?

At first you may want to tell no-one. The fact that you have cancer, even if the outlook for the future is good, may feel like very private information and not something you want to share. Who you decide to tell personally must, of course, be your decision, but you are likely to include:

- close family members;
- close friends;
- your employer, if appropriate.

Basically, those people who you are closest to and who will be most affected by your cancer. The process of contacting people may take some time: devoting whole days to speaking with your family and friends is unlikely to feel like an easy option. Explaining the details of your diagnosis is a draining and emotional experience, and while many people will want to spend a lot of time with you or talking on the phone, you may want to keep your conversations quite short. You may also start to feel that you have related your story so many times that you can't bear to have the same conversation yet again. Don't rush the process, and consider who you want to see personally, who you can contact by phone, and who you can write to: this will help to spread the workload.

News travels fast, and you may find that your wider circle of friends, acquaintances, colleagues and so on become aware of your cancer sooner than you expect. If you want to restrict the news only to those people you tell personally, then do not be afraid to ask them to treat it confidentially, and explain to them that you do not yet feel ready to tell the world at large.

Assuming you are well enough to be mobile and go out of the house, you cannot avoid meeting people – neighbours, acquaintances, contacts – who do not know about your cancer. When people ask how you are, it can be difficult to know what to say: Should you deflect the situation and not tell them, or do you say, 'Not too good – I've got cancer'? Your reaction will probably vary depending on how you feel that day. Remember that the most important person in this situation is you, and you are not under any obligation to pass on the details of your cancer to all and sundry if you do not want to.

Inevitably, tricky situations will arise when you meet people who are not aware of your cancer and who comment, for example, on your physical appearance. It may be that you lose your hair temporarily while undergoing chemotherapy and an acquaintance comments on your 'dramatic haircut', or on the fact that you have lost weight or don't look as well as when they last saw you. Comments like these are not intended to be malicious or hurtful, but they can cause distress. Most people are deeply embarrassed and upset when told the actual reason for your bald head or your weight loss – if you choose to tell them. There is no formula for dealing with these situations, but it does become easier as you become more accustomed to talking about your cancer.

When and how to tell?

Telling close family and friends

There is also no easy way to tell the people close to you that you have cancer, and you may want to ask your wife or partner, a member of your family or a close friend to help you if you find it difficult to cope alone. It might be helpful to start by making a list of those people you want to speak to personally rather than allowing them to hear the news 'on the grapevine'. You can't rehearse your conversations, but you can decide in advance the important facts you want to convey, such as:

- what type of cancer you have;
- what type of treatment is proposed for you;
- how well or unwell you feel at the moment;
- whether you will be staying in hospital;
- an indication of the likely prognosis, if you know;
- whether there are any specific matters you would like help with (lifts to the hospital, help at home, walking the dog, company, etc).

Finding the right time to tell people depends on when you feel ready, and it can be made more difficult by the fact that you find talking about your cancer very upsetting or awkward. You may also feel that you already have enough to deal with, without the added distress of coping with other people's reactions. However, putting it off means that you continue to have one more source of worry on your mind. You may even find that after the distress of the initial conversation, you find some relief in starting to talk more openly. Sadly, pretending to the outside world that it doesn't exist will not make it go away, although there may be situations where you do delay breaking the news – if a friend or relative has an important exam or a big celebration or a holiday which you don't want to disrupt. It is your choice, and you must do what feels right to you.

Whether you break the news face to face or by telephone, try to make sure that you have enough time to talk, and that you will not be interrupted or distracted. Perhaps ask, 'Do you have time for a chat?' This will often act as a signal that you have something important to say, but it will help if you also make it clear that you have a serious matter to discuss. You might say, for example, 'You might have realized that I haven't been too well recently', or simply, 'I'm afraid I've got some bad news'. It is tempting to try to soften your words or to play down your situation to make it less distressing for the recipient of your news, but it is important not to avoid giving them the facts.

Our first instinct was to cling on to each other and tell no-one. We

66

realized, though, that this was not a situation we could conceal for long, even if we wanted to. It was further complicated by the fact that we were running a business together, and we didn't want our clients to worry that they would no longer be properly looked after! In the event we began telling close family and friends very quickly but we were still in shock and deeply upset and had no idea how to go about having these conversations. As time passed, it became a little easier as we got used to the new medical vocabulary and hit upon phrases to start our conversations: 'Please don't panic, but we've got some bad news', 'I'm afraid we're having a bit of a crisis'. It all sounds very obvious, but there are times when you simply cannot find any words to describe what's happening except, 'I've got cancer'.

There is no easy or euphemistic way to say, 'I've got cancer'. Most people react with shock and horror when they hear the word 'cancer', and immediately assume the worst, particularly if they are a close family member or friend. You may not feel like going into details yourself, and if you have someone with you, they can help at this stage of the conversation by providing some basic factual information, or a brief chronology of the events that led up to your diagnosis. Perhaps you can start the conversation, then say, 'I'm finding this very difficult to talk about at the moment. Do you mind talking to (your wife/partner/mother/friend) instead?' It may be that the outlook for the future is good, and you can give some reassurance about the anticipated effectiveness of treatment, for example. If this is not the case, then you need to make equally sure this is understood: 'I'm afraid it sounds serious'.

It is almost impossible to have such a conversation and not become emotional, and it is important for you not to feel awkward about expressing your feelings as well as the facts about your cancer. You *are* allowed to say, 'Right now, I feel really scared' or 'I still feel completely shell-shocked'.

These conversations can be upsetting, and depending on who you are talking to, you may want to keep it quite short in the first instance. You can suggest talking again later in the day or the following day. Just as it was difficult for you to absorb information about your cancer through the shock of diagnosis, so it can be hard for loved ones to do the same. It is important that they appreciate the seriousness of what you are telling them, so keeping the details reasonably brief and factual will make them easier to absorb. Close family and friends may well want to spend a lot of time with you when they hear about your diagnosis, talking about your cancer with you and showing their support.

Telling children about your cancer can be especially painful, as we instinctively want to protect them from something as unpleasant as cancer. Trying to conceal the truth from your own child or others who are close to you is rarely a good idea. They need time to come to terms with your illness too, and it is not fair to deny them that time in the belief that you are shielding them from something they can't understand. Finding the right words to explain your cancer to children may take time, and you will also need to allow them time to ask their own questions. Try to answer them as honestly as you can in terms they can grasp, be aware of how well they are absorbing what you tell them and don't necessarily assume that older children will understand or cope with the news better than younger ones, or vice versa. They may want to repeat their questions to make sure they have understood, so try not to be too impatient if you have to go through your explanations several times or reiterate your assurances that your cancer is in no way their fault. The cancer support organization BACUP publishes a booklet called *What Do I Tell the Children?*, which might help you to find the right words.

You will repeat your news a number of times, and have similar conversations with a number of different people. You may become tired of using the same words and describing the same sequence of events over and over again, not to mention coping with all the various reactions people display. This can become tiring and frustrating at a time when you need to devote your physical and emotional energies to your own well-being. It might be a good idea to ask a few close friends if they would mind passing on the news to other friends, or for one family member to inform certain others. Don't feel that you have to shoulder all the responsibility yourself. Alternatively, a short letter might be appropriate for passing on the news to certain people, if this is what you want to do.

Telling your employer

Although the emotional ties to people like your employer and work colleagues may be less strong, this does not mean that telling them about your cancer is any easier for you.

If you are in employment you will need to tell your employer about your cancer and make sure arrangements are worked out for you to take time off for your treatment. There may also be times when you feel too unwell to work, and your employer needs to appreciate that you will not necessarily be able to predict these in advance. You may fear that your employer will not view the prospect of regular or prolonged absences from work favourably. However, they are more likely to be distressed about your cancer than worried about any disruption that may arise at work. Most employers should be sympathetic to working out flexible arrangements which accommodate your treatment and illness, and this is discussed further in Chapter 7.

Dealing with reactions to your cancer

Telling people about your cancer is difficult, and you will be prepared to expect that. What can be unexpectedly exhausting is dealing with people's reactions to the news. It is natural to be concerned about how your close family and friends will be affected, and we all dread passing on bad news and the reactions we know will result. Different people react in different ways, and although you are the person who needs most support at this time, there will also be a period when you have to field a variety of responses to your news.

We were initially unprepared for people's reactions too – everyone wanted to jump in the car and come to visit, to support and help us, and just to be close. But when people ask on the phone, it's hard to make your brain work at all, let alone figure out whether or not you want visitors. In time, we could anticipate people's reactions – 'Can I do anything?' and 'Can I come and see you?' – and had thought out in advance our own reactions: 'Could you just keep in touch by phone?' 'Could you phone tomorrow and perhaps visit then?'; 'Could you collect a prescription while we're at the hospital?'; 'Could you pass on the news to X?' It took time to reach the stage where we were thinking clearly and could be specific, but gradually we got there.

Your close family and friends are likely to react at first with shock and disbelief. Comments like, 'You seemed so well last time we saw you' or 'But you always seemed so strong and healthy' express how difficult serious illness is to accept. Although people are aware that many cancers are completely undiscriminating in whom they affect, they still find it hard to believe that someone close to them could be affected – cancer always happens to someone else. A common knee-jerk reaction is to deny your cancer: 'That can't be right' or 'I can't believe it'. You should be prepared for anger too, once the initial shock has passed – those close to you will feel rage that this should happen to *you*. This anger may feel as if it is directed at you personally, and can be difficult to cope with. You can do nothing to make your cancer disappear (which is what we would all like, of course), and other people's anger can feel very unkind and unjustified, as if they are accusing you of choosing to have cancer. Such outbursts can be very painful, but many people do need to express their anger as a form of emotional release.

In some ways more difficult are those who are completely unable to cope with the fact of your cancer, and who react as though nothing has happened. You are trying to convey a very serious piece of news, and it can be both disconcerting and upsetting if the sole reaction is, 'Sorry to hear that, mate. I suppose you won't be coming to the pub on Friday?' Many men do find illness and the emotions it generates very hard to talk about, and therefore feel it is better to say nothing at all. This does not mean that the emotional reaction is any less powerful, but rather that the vocabulary and the confidence to express those emotions are suppressed. Reactions such as, 'Nothing I say will get rid of the cancer, so why bother' or 'I wouldn't know what to say – I leave that to my wife' can seem uncaring but this is rarely the reality. It is more likely that your friend or relative simply has no idea what to say and is so embarrassed at the prospect of any emotional reaction that they try to continue as normal and treat you as if your cancer doesn't exist.

People can also be uncertain about how to talk to you or mistakenly feel that you have enough to cope with and that it is better not to 'bother' you at all. This doesn't mean that they don't care or are not interested in what is happening, but rather that they don't want to add to your problems: 'He's got enough on his plate without me visiting/phoning' or 'I'd call, but I just don't know what to say'. What feels to you like a withdrawal of support or friendship is often no more than confusion about how to behave. It can be useful to make it clear to friends and family that you would welcome

70

their phone calls or visits, but that they should not be offended if sometimes you are not feeling strong enough or simply in the right mood to chat or see people. They will understand, and will probably welcome any such guidance you can give them.

Although you are still the same person, it can be difficult to accept that some people will treat you in a different way after hearing of your cancer. Being considered a cancer patient first and 'Neil' second can be intensely frustrating, especially if you are making efforts to retain as much control over your situation as you can. People may treat you as though you are no longer capable of your usual activities and try to take control of tasks or situations which you are perfectly able to manage yourself. They will have the very best intentions, but may need to be reminded that while you appreciate their concern, it would be better if they waited until you *really* need their help.

Being treated as a different person can manifest itself in more subtle ways. Most of us have a perception of ourselves which is associated with strength in some form, be it

- as a breadwinner;
- in relation to our family;
- as an achiever;
- as someone who always copes;
- as the person who always sorts out practical problems at home;
- in a purely physical sense;

and this perception is often shared by those around you. In the same way that physical illness can undermine your own sense of strength, so others may see you in a new light. People may feel that they should no longer rely on you for your 'strong' qualities, not so much because they no longer exist but because you have something more important to concentrate on – your health and treatment. This can also be reflected in how they talk to you, and can be frustrating because you still need to be involved in the day-to-day problems and irritations of people's lives. People might think, 'We won't bother to tell him about that, we'll just sort it out ourselves.'

As a man, it can be confusing and distressing to realize that the expectations connected with your 'strong' qualities which were previously placed on you – both by yourself and others – have changed. On the one hand, people want to look after and 'mother' you, to take control on your behalf and ensure that you are not worried or bothered by the trivia of everyday life. On the other hand, you may also find that those close to you, in an effort to prevent you from becoming withdrawn, urge you to 'pull yourself together' or not to 'let it get you down'. The very fact that people are reacting differently to you points to a change in their expectations which you may find difficult to deal with at first.

Although men are increasingly encouraged not to bottle up their emotions, there may still exist an unvoiced expectation that you will find the strength and reserves to cope simply because you are a man. This can feel deeply unfair because you just can't win! You are urged to talk, to open up, to discuss your feelings but you may sense a slight discomfort in those around you that you need to, especially if this is uncharacteristic behaviour for you. If you keep your feelings to yourself, loved ones become concerned that you are trying to be too strong for them. Perhaps the best course is simply to trust to instinct and to talk to those you trust and feel comfortable with.

In the very early stages, you may not have the emotional energy to take as much interest in the trivia of everyday life as usual. Later, however, it can be very important to feel that you are not being sidelined because you are no longer capable of any useful input into other people's problems. To be told after the event that 'We didn't think you'd be interested/didn't want to upset you/thought you had enough to worry about' can be very isolating. Although you need extra support, you don't want to be constantly handled with kid gloves. It will take some time for you, together with your family and friends, to reach a good balance, but in the meantime you can assure them that staying in touch with the everyday details of other people's lives is more helpful than troublesome for you.

Although I became very unwell very quickly, I still needed to feel involved in – and preferably in control over – the practical changes which we needed to make to our lives, and to a large extent, we managed this with the support of family and friends. What became extremely frustrating was to hear some people, with the best of intentions, asking Helen about my cancer and how I was rather than asking me – the classic scenario of talking about 'the patient' as if he isn't there. These people were presumably trying to save me the effort and potential distress of going through my story yet again. Of course, there were times when I didn't feel like talking, but on the whole, it feels better to be given the option! Similarly, while there were occasions when other people's news felt pretty irrelevant, it was infinitely preferable to being excluded from all 'normal' conversation.

Making it easier for others

After the initial shock of your diagnosis has receded, you may begin to feel the pressures of making it easier for other people to talk to you and come to terms with your cancer. It is natural for all of us to feel upset at hearing bad news and worrying about how to react, and you may find that you play down your situation to ease other people's concern and distress. You may find yourself reassuring your family and friends that, for example, you are not in any pain or discomfort, that treatment is considered very effective or that you are receiving very high quality care in an excellent hospital. Your conversations might give the impression that you are feeling much more positive and upbeat than you actually feel, even if your situation is very serious. People obviously prefer to hear good news (although not as much as you!), and the pressure to assure them that you are feeling 'fine' in spite of everything can be emotionally tiring.

In many cases, you will also have to take the lead in talking about your cancer and treatment, as people can be reticent about asking for details, however much they want to know all that is happening to you. Most of us are very ignorant about cancer and its treatments until someone close to us is affected, and therefore we simply don't know what questions to ask or how to start talking. Describing your cancer or talking about how your treatment works can be very beneficial in prompting questions. For example, most people who have not had contact with chemotherapy or radiotherapy find it impossible to visualize how the treatment is given, and are also unlikely to know what it is. They will probably feel too embarrassed to ask you such a basic question, so describing how it is administered and what it 'looks like' can help them to understand more about what you are going through.

However much you take pleasure in talking to your family and friends, don't underestimate how emotionally tiring it can be to chat about your cancer. Remember that there will be times when you don't feel like talking, and a hug or watching TV or listening to music or just sitting quietly with your companion is all you can manage. You don't have to 'entertain' people, even if you do feel some responsibility to do so.

Feeling a need to be 'strong' for the benefit of others can be draining too. There will be times when you exaggerate how well you feel or how much energy you have so that others will worry less. After a gathering of friends or a family meal, for example, you may find you are exhausted from the effort of keeping up a strong front. You might look forward to a visit from a friend and feel you must be positive and cheerful so that they can enjoy the visit too, and aren't left with an image of you as tired and unwell. We naturally want to feel that our family and friends enjoy our company, so we make a particular effort to be a good companion. Just don't overdo it!

6

Personal relationships

As we know, cancer is not a disease which can be treated quickly and simply and then forgotten. One man whose daughter had cancer treatment as a baby described it as 'lifetime membership of a club'. Although his daughter is now in her teens and completely well, the experience has never faded entirely and a slight fear of recurrence always remains in the back of his mind. His feelings are very typical. Some cancers do respond extremely well to treatment and some men are completely cured, but the check-ups can continue for years, so that you never forget completely.

It is a powerful experience which leaves a lasting impression and which can bring about changes in your outlook, priorities and lifestyle. Many men comment during or after their treatment that 'I could never have gone through it without my wife/partner/parents/ friend' or 'The treatment was unpleasant, but I wanted to get through it for the sake of my children/wife etc'. Comments like these emphasize how much we value and rely on our family and friends, often unconsciously, and how important these relationships become at times of crisis. You may find it difficult at first to accept that you need their support, especially if you have always been – and been seen as – a strong and supportive person yourself. There will be difficult and distressing times, but you will find your journey through treatment easier to bear if you undertake it *together* with the people you are close to.

This does not mean that you will not have some rocky times and sticky moments together with your loved ones. It is often assumed that people facing a crisis together will automatically 'pull together' and be constantly mutually supportive and saintly. It is true that for some people, facing a crisis together does strengthen their relationship. Others find their relationship under a huge strain. There is no 'norm' and no one should be expected to live up to unrealistic ideals of behaviour. However, if you stick together with those close to you and are willing to accept that we are all only human, then you may be surprised at the level of support you are able to offer each other.

Your reactions

While you are experiencing the initial shock of diagnosis it can be hard to put your thoughts into words. You and those close to you may find that you are too dazed to talk much, your thoughts are racing and confused and you experience a whole range of emotions which are not easy to express. Anger and fear may be among these, and it can be difficult to find the right words to tell people how you feel, beyond 'I just feel so angry – why me?' or 'I'm so frightened about what's going to happen'. In time, your thoughts will become clearer and it will help to share them with someone close to you, someone you trust to really *listen* to what you are saying and who will support you by giving you time to talk when you need to.

Anger

It is common to feel anger and rage that cancer has been inflicted on you. You want to shout 'Why me? What have I done to deserve this?' while knowing that there is no 'good' answer. You can read technical explanations about how cancers develop, or the factors which make us more susceptible but this is not really the point. All you want is for someone to tell you it's been a ghastly mistake, and that in fact you have a perfectly straightforward and treatable condition.

> We were almost too numb to be angry at first, and oddly, what anger we did feel was directed at the small but (to us) significant inadequacies of the health system. There is also the suspicion that if you once let go of your emotions, you'll never be able to stop and can wave goodbye to any last semblance of control and rational thought. We were trying desperately hard to be calm and sensible although we were at times incredibly frustrated at the apparent lack of action or progress and at our own powerlessness. There was also the sense that everything we'd worked so hard for years to build up was crumbling around us and that our whole future together was disappearing before our eyes.

We generally consider anger to be a negative emotion, but it can have a positive side in helping you to focus your thoughts and energy. You can channel your anger in a constructive way so that rather than saying, 'It's not fair', you gradually come to think, 'OK, so I've got cancer. I can't change that but I can fight to cope with it the best way I can.' When talking about serious illness, and especially cancer, we often use language which we associate with a battle – 'I'm not going to let this disease beat me', 'I'm going to fight this with all my strength'. Cancer becomes the 'enemy', to be treated as something which has to be fought with every possible resource. You can draw on your anger to fuel your determination and a more positive frame of mind which will help you to face your cancer and treatment with greater strength.

Inevitably, frustrations can simmer inside you and there will be times when these boil over and your anger is directed at the people you love most. This is rarely because you feel angry with them personally, but because it is natural to express your emotions to those closest to you. If your anger stems from the sudden loss of control over your destiny, from a sense of loss of strength and 'status' or a sudden feeling of inadequacy, it can be hard to put these feelings into a coherent explanation – and you may not feel like doing so. However supportive those close to you are, they need some understanding of your anger in order not to feel hurt and shut out. Of course, you won't feel like entering into lengthy explanations every time you snap at someone, but if communication is good, people will have a basic understanding of why you feel so frustrated and find it easier to offer you the right type of support when you need it.

It can come as a surprise to experience anger at what is intended as kindness by others. For example, acquaintances who have a friend or relation who has been treated for cancer may say to you, 'I know how you feel. My friend's friend had cancer, and it was awful.' It may seem to you that they claim to know exactly what you are going through, having shared a similar experience only second-hand. You may feel enraged because nobody knows exactly what is in your mind except you. Everybody's experience of cancer is different, and even two cancer patients talking to one another can't know exactly what is in each other's mind. Cancer patients are still individuals even if bound by a shared disease! However, we all draw on our own experiences in our conversations, and people will try to sympathize with your situation by remembering how they felt in similar circumstances, either first or second-hand. The comparisons are well meant, even if you feel like shouting at them, 'You haven't got a clue what it's like!'

In a similar vein, there is a fine line between sympathy and patronizing behaviour. You might find that people are more tactile than usual with you and, for example, touch your arm frequently when talking to you. They are probably trying to demonstrate physically their support and sympathy for you, showing that they are close to you – but it can feel very patronizing. Pregnant women sometimes complain that when their pregnancy becomes obvious, even casual acquaintances feel they have some right to touch their 'bump', as if it has become public property. This is a similar syndrome, and it's difficult to avoid without causing offence: you might feel like saying, 'Please don't touch me, I'm not a cat', but at the same time don't want to convey any sense of rejection.

You can hardly avoid changes in your perspective on life following your diagnosis. What used to cause your blood to boil with anger and frustration may seem irrelevant now and people who moan endlessly about their seemingly trivial problems can become a further source of irritation to you. A friend who complains of toothache or of standing in the supermarket queue for ages or the breakdown of their car may leave you feeling, 'I wish I had your problems' or 'Think yourself lucky!' It is difficult not to voice these thoughts or to be angry with others for taking for granted aspects of life which are currently beyond your reach. Your sense of perspective and outlook on life have taken a battering. In the meantime it is helpful if others take account of this, but life is not that simple and you will need your reserves of patience.

Some men find that anger, whether a brief but violent outburst or a simmering, seething frustration, is expressed in unexpected and uncharacteristic ways. You may be more prone than usual to sudden outbursts or a tendency to snap unreasonably for little or no reason. You may feel a need to exert your authority more than usual, to 'prove' that you are still the same strong, capable man, to insist that things are done 'your' way, or become more defensive about your role and abilities. The temptation may be strong to reject ungraciously and crossly offers of help with a task which is traditionally 'yours', such as walking the dog or cutting the grass.

If you are usually mild-mannered and even-tempered, experiencing anger and frustration from a variety of sources may come as a shock, both to you and your family. This is not a reason to suppress it as 'inappropriate' behaviour. You *are* allowed to be angry, and without feeling guilty or the need to apologize afterwards.

Fear

Any step into unknown territory holds fears. Starting college or a new job, moving house and visiting the dentist all cause us a degree of fear either because we don't know what to expect from the experience and/or because we anticipate that it will be unpleasant. Dealing with cancer is certainly a league ahead in terms of the intensity of our fears, but the root cause is the same: fear of the unknown. There are so many unknown factors involved that our security is profoundly threatened:

• Will I be in pain?
• What is the treatment like?
• Will the treatment hurt?
• Will the treatment work?
• What does the future hold for me?
• How will my family cope?
• Will my life ever be 'normal' again?
• How will I manage to get through this?

Becoming well-informed about your cancer and treatment can help to allay certain fears: the greater your knowledge and understanding of what is happening, the more control you can take and the less uncertainty you will feel about specific aspects of your disease or treatment. However, fear is not a logical emotion and a theoretical understanding will not always prevent you from worrying. It cannot necessarily help you with more general fears – about coping or about the future, for example.

One of the aspects of cancer and its treatment which causes most fear is uncertainty: uncertainty at how effective your treatment is and uncertainty at how much of your cancer will be eradicated. Waiting for the results of X-rays or blood tests, perhaps not hearing anything for several weeks between treatments, can cause great anxiety. You don't know what to prepare yourself for or what plans to make, you can't stop thinking about what might or might not happen. Tension is bound to build up, however much you try to take your mind off your cancer.

After the first awful month or six weeks, it was clear that I was responding well to my chemotherapy. Following so much bad

79

news, this was more than we could have hoped for. But there was still a very long way to go and although my tumour markers were moving in the right direction, there was no guarantee that this would continue. We anticipated each hospital visit (weekly at this stage) with a mixture of unvoiced hope and stomach-turning trepidation. Butterflies? Legions of them, all on overtime. If the details were not immediately forthcoming, it took a huge effort of will to ask, 'What are my tumour markers this week?' or 'What did the CT scan show?'

Apart from immediate fears about the possible unpleasantness of treatment, thinking about the future is likely to emerge as your single greatest fear. This can encompass a whole range of ideas, from 'How will I manage to get through my treatment?' to 'Will I ever get better?' At times when you are feeling physically low, you might wonder if you can bear to undergo any more treatment or how you can possibly tolerate the effects of your cancer any longer. How will you cope if you become physically incapacitated in some way? Who will look after you? How will you manage financially? Do you fear that your family and friends will eventually tire of supporting you and that you will feel a burden to them?

Fighting against cancer shakes the very foundations of your life, and it would be unusual not to experience fears that your life is toppling around you. These thought processes cannot be banished, but you can help to keep them in perspective by sharing them with someone you trust to take you seriously and listen. There may be times when you know your fears are irrational, but you need someone to take the time to talk them through with you. You may not expect solutions to your fears, but sharing them and knowing that someone you like and respect acknowledges and appreciates your worries can make them more bearable.

Just to hear someone say, 'Of course you're not being stupid! I can see now how difficult this is for you' or 'I hadn't appreciated until now how cancer takes over your life' can be enormously helpful and will help you to realize that you don't have to face your fears alone.

Sometimes a desire to express anxiety can be inhibited by a superstitious worry that voicing fears will somehow make them come true. For example, you are anxious that your treatment might not be as effective as you'd hoped, but you daren't say so because you don't want to 'tempt fate'. We know this cannot happen but it can still make us hold back from saying all we want to. Even sharing this fear can help. Nobody will think you foolish: others are likely to admit to exactly the same worry.

If you spend a lot of time alone, your fears are more likely to become magnified. Similarly, if you are not sleeping well, fears can get out of control in the middle of the night. It would be foolish to pretend that they can be avoided completely, but it is important not to allow them to take over your mind. Sharing your worries will help. It is tempting to be 'strong' and keep them to yourself, but the people around you will be aware of your state of mind and will want to help. It is, however, important to remember that there may be occasions when you simply prefer to maintain a 'stiff upper lip'. There are times when this can be an equally valid coping mechanism.

Attitude

The prospect of dealing with your cancer and treatment can feel like an insurmountable burden, so that you just don't know how to begin 'coping' with this new experience. You might be very withdrawn and wrapped up in your thoughts at the beginning, feeling very isolated and believing that nobody can understand what you are going through. This is a natural reaction, and true of any catastrophe – it is difficult to accept that anyone has ever experienced similar feelings and that you are not completely alone in this situation. It can be made more painful by the fact that up to a point, life around you has to continue as normal. Children need attention, dogs need walking, you still have to (try to) eat and sleep, the world goes on functioning around you. You may have deep fears about the future, yet find it hard to accept that your life has been threatened.

Your mental attitude can help you as you progress through your treatment. Although there is no medical evidence that a positive attitude will make any difference to the success of your treatment, it can help you to feel stronger about coping with your treatment and its side-effects and to take pleasure in those aspects of your everyday life which are still 'normal'.

For some people, positive thinking comes naturally and they attack their cancer with the same vigour and determination they demonstrate in all areas of their life. For many others though, it is not a natural state of mind – perhaps you feel resigned to your cancer and take a stoical attitude, dealing with each day as it comes without actually making up your mind to fight the disease. For some men, trying not to be negative takes a huge effort, and there may be a danger of slipping into depression. This is a serious condition and it can affect your entire life, but it can be treated successfully with anti-depressant drugs. It is not uncommon among cancer patients, and is certainly not a condition which you should suffer in silence, even if you do feel awkward about approaching the subject.

Even if you have a basically positive attitude towards fighting your cancer, there will be times when you feel very low, and wonder whether there is any point in going through unpleasant treatments or putting up any fight at all. Everyone has periods when they feel overwhelmed by their cancer and wonder if they have the energy and will to battle against it any longer. Of course, it is impossible to feel positive all the time and it is very important not to feel guilty when you feel miserable and low. There will be days when you feel that you just don't care any more, that you can't be bothered to make any more effort. If your treatment is not progressing as well as you had hoped, you might think, 'There's nothing I can do, so what have I got to feel positive about?' At the same time, you might feel that you should put on a brave face for the benefit of family or friends. While this is bound to occur from time to time, it won't help you to suppress your real feelings constantly – you *do* need someone to share your emotions with, to talk to, shout at and cry with.

In fact, as your treatment gets underway, you may feel a sense of relief that something is happening, and that you are no longer in limbo. Unexpectedly for many people, cancer wards and out-patient clinics are not the grim and gloomy places one might expect, so if you have been dreading your visits, especially as an in-patient, you may find this less gruelling than you had anticipated. In spite of that, you are bound to experience fears about how effectively your treatment is working, and look forward with trepidation to each X-ray or blood test which provides information about your progress. Some days you may feel physically good and mentally positive, and other days weak and unwell and miserable. During your journey through treatment, you will experience many emotions, some of which may be new to you or have been suppressed for years. They are all perfectly valid even if you feel foolish for being unusually 'emotional'.

Loss of control

You may spend days when you feel completely powerless to do anything – the loss of control over what is happening to your body can make you feel that the same has happened to the rest of your life. Most of us are not doctors, let alone cancer specialists, so our ignorance about the disease and its treatment contributes to our sense of helplessness. We can learn a certain amount from books and leaflets, but we still remain in the dark in terms of understanding exactly what is happening and why.

If you are also feeling physically low, this can make you feel even more helpless. If you have previously worked but are now too ill to do so, or you led an active life with regular commitments which you can no longer fulfil, the sense that your life is out of your control can be cruelly emphasized. It may be that you need help with personal tasks you could manage perfectly easily before, and you fear becoming increasingly dependent on your family or nursing staff for basic necessities. Living with cancer can take considerable adjustment.

How can you maintain some control over your life when you feel that events and other people are taking over? It is hard to accept that you need more help and support than before, especially if you are usually very independent. You can start by trying to become well-informed about your treatment and progress, and you can still take decisions for yourself. Let your family and friends know that your cancer does not mean that you can no longer think for yourself, even if sometimes you can't muster the enthusiasm even to decide between chips or mashed potatoes! Although there may be times when you feel too ill to be interested in what is happening around you, it is important for you to feel that you are still treated as an individual, and not just a cancer patient.

Managing together

You may find 'opening up' to your close family and friends about your cancer extremely difficult at first. The whole experience feels very private and personal – after all, it is *your* life at stake – and you may feel ambivalent about the sudden increase in people who want to visit you and share the experience. Whether or not yours is a close family, they will want to feel involved and make their support known to you. Friends are likely to react similarly.

It will help you to cope better if you don't feel completely alone, and it can make a big difference to make a positive decision to cope together. In fact, simply sitting down quietly with a close relative or friend – whoever will be spending most time with you – and saying, 'This is going to be tough, but we'll get through it together' can be a morale booster. Knowing that you are not alone, that you have support when you need it and that someone else is fighting *with* you, is very comforting.

We'd spent the past five years working together and were used to spending a lot of our time with each other and dealing with issues together. We thought we were a pretty good team! But this was completely new territory, and we didn't really have a clue where to begin. We'd never had much to do with the health service, so that was all new to us. I was fast becoming too ill to take much of an active role in the various practical issues that needed sorting out, but we sat down and talked through what needed to be done, and with some crucial help from family and friends, we got on with it – because that's what we'd always done. Even then, I don't think we realized the extent of what we were facing (which was probably just as well!), but we clung to our gut feeling that if we stuck together and didn't give in, we'd somehow manage to grope our way through these black days. At times, it felt like the two of us against the world but we were determined to 'manage' somehow.

Even if you are in a reasonably positive frame of mind, there will be bad times. It is important for you to have someone to talk to and, when you need to, to depend on. This may be your wife/partner, mother/father, brother/sister, son/daughter or a close friend. Who they are is less important than their role in your current situation. Although there will be times when you feel completely solitary, you will need someone to share your thoughts with. You may have different people you talk to in different circumstances. You might find that you prefer to talk to certain people when you are feeling positive as they are good at bolstering your cheerful state of mind. There may be others who are especially helpful and sympathetic when you feel low or angry. The important point is that you do not stew in your own thoughts and fears alone. Communication is vital and you do need a 'talking partner', someone to talk with you about the ups and downs of living with your cancer.

It is important for those close to you to be aware of how you feel, and you can help them by being specific when you are asked, 'How are you feeling today?' Saying, 'I'm not too bad' or 'Struggling on' doesn't give people much information to act on. Once you have become attuned to any side-effects of your cancer or chemotherapy or radiotherapy treatment, make sure your family are aware of them. For example, they will be aware of the importance to your overall well-being of maintaining a reasonable diet, and may be encouraging you to eat or trying to find the foods which are most tempting for you. If you feel particularly nauseous on certain days and find it difficult to eat much, then making this clear rather than just saying 'I don't feel like eating' will help them to understand. The best way for you to manage together is to keep communicating and sharing information. If communication is working well, then even when you are feeling that you can't be bothered to make the effort or are feeling low and just want to snap, 'Don't fuss!', those around you will have a better understanding of your reasons and will be better placed to offer you constructive help.

In a slightly different vein, you will also have to field questions from family and friends about how your treatment is progressing. You might prefer to divulge very little and employ stalling tactics: 'It'll be a while before we know how well I'm responding'; or you may be happy to share more detailed information. Remember that most people have little understanding of how cancer treatments are monitored (by blood tests, scans, etc) or how long it can take before any conclusions about your progress are reached. You may find you have numerous similar conversations, trying to explain the mechanics of your treatment. More annoying are comments like, 'You're looking so well, it must be working' from people who have no idea how you really are. Others may be afraid that you won't want to talk at all, so don't ask about your progress but chatter on any subject *except* your cancer. You may have to take the lead if you do want to talk about it.

Living with your cancer is hard for your family too, and there will be times when those closest to you find it difficult to sustain the level of support they want to offer, however willing they may be. The whole experience is physically and emotionally draining for them too, and they also need to be 'allowed' to say, 'This isn't fair. I can't bear it.' At times like this you may feel a terrible responsibility for their distress. Remember always that they are not blaming you, and that sharing these feelings will ultimately help you all to cope better than bottling them up.

As a society, we are uncomfortable about discussing serious or life-threatening illness, and cancer is still something of a taboo subject. We often don't know how to broach the subject and prefer to avoid it altogether rather than saying 'the wrong thing'. We are also afraid of upsetting 'the patient' by mentioning their condition, when in fact all parties would be much relieved by an open and honest conversation. To add to the difficulty, many men find it hard to express their emotions, especially if they have been brought up and conditioned by society to be strong and dependable, not showing any unmanly 'weakness'.

If you are not accustomed to talking about your feelings, it can be hard to find both the vocabulary and the confidence to express how you feel. Perhaps there is a fear that you will be told to 'pull yourself together' or 'be a man' – or a sense that you should do this automatically, and shouldn't need support. Starting to talk is the most difficult part, even with someone you are close to. If you don't know where to begin, you could try saying something general – 'I'm having a bad day today' or 'This is more difficult than I'd expected' – to start your conversation. Nobody will laugh at you or think badly of you – they are more likely to feel concerned that they haven't been able to offer you enough time or the type of support you need. There will be times when you don't feel the need or the desire to talk, but want to be left alone with your private thoughts. This should be respected, but don't feel that this must be the norm.

Equally, it can be hard to take the plunge if those around you treat you as a man who 'keeps his feelings to himself' and aren't aware that you need an outlet for your thoughts and worries. It can be very isolating to feel too reticent to make the first move and leave you feeling very alone. If you do feel alone, or if for other reasons you are not able to draw on family and friends for support, do mention this to the medical staff treating you or to your GP. You may feel foolish and have difficulty finding the right words – you may not want to say, 'I need someone to talk to.' Your doctors will understand that coping with cancer is not just a matter of treatment, that your state of mind is also important. You could try saying instead, 'This is hard to say, but I'm feeling a bit low and I'd like to have a chat about things.' Perhaps you can say the same to a family member or friend, in person or on the phone. If you wish, your GP can arrange for you to speak to a counsellor or put you in touch with a support group (see later in this chapter). The first step is always the hardest to take, and it takes courage, but it will make a difference to your state of mind to feel that you are *not* alone.

You won't always feel like seeing visitors or chatting to people on the phone, however much you may value their support. It can be difficult to say this without fearing that people will feel rejected, and won't offer again. Your family and friends will understand if you tell them, 'I'd like to see you, but I'm afraid I'm not feeling so good at the moment. Perhaps you could phone next week when I should be feeling stronger.' Alternatively you can warn visitors that while they are very welcome, their visits may have to be short: 'It's always good to see you, but I'm sure you'll understand if I'm not up to a long visit.'

Visitors or phone calls will also be valuable in keeping you in touch with other people's lives. It is natural to become very wrapped up in your disease and treatment because of the fundamental change it has brought to your life. There will be times when hearing your friends' news or details from colleagues about what is happening at work seems completely irrelevant and pointless to you, and you just don't want to know. It can be very refreshing though, to listen to relatively trivial information and news as a means of keeping in touch and maintaining a sense of normality in your life. You may find after such a conversation that you feel brighter and more aware.

If you are spending time in hospital, people generally assume that you would welcome visitors to help pass the time. This is not true for everyone – when you are undergoing treatment and feeling vulnerable, you might feel: 'I don't want people to see me like this' and prefer to restrict your visitors to your close family or particular friends. Again, you may fear that people will feel offended if you reject their offers to visit you in hospital, but they will understand and respect your feelings.

For the first few weeks, I couldn't bear anyone but Helen to visit me in hospital. I had become very weak very quickly and I just didn't want anyone else to see me like this – painfully thin, hair falling out all over the pillow, barely able to walk. Even my parents were barred at first although we kept in touch daily with phone calls from the hospital. Later in my treatment when I had regained weight and was much stronger, I was still reluctant to have visitors in hospital other than Helen and a few others. On the whole I preferred to keep my treatment and social contact with friends quite separate – which does not mean at all that I did not value their visits and support! We found other ways to pass the time instead, much of which revolved around the TV – I remember this as the 'summer of sport' – the football of Euro 96, tennis at Wimbledon, as much cricket as I could find.

Changes in relationships

Even if you normally regard yourself as a 'strong' person, it is natural in these circumstances to turn to your wife or partner or a member of your family for extra support. At heart you will want to remain in control as much as possible, but you are unlikely to want to handle all the practical details of, say, hospital appointments and your treatment single-handed. You may look to, for example, your wife to be strong and capable in communicating with your hospital and doctors. Initially, this can present difficulties on two counts. First, it can be hard to accept that you want to opt out of a degree of control of your situation. Second, it may be that the person from whom you are seeking that support finds it difficult to give because they are also profoundly affected by your diagnosis. They too may want to be strong for you, but simply feel incapable of taking charge in the very early days. Tensions can result from the resulting sense of helplessness you might feel at first, but do allow yourselves time to absorb what has happened before trying to adapt your lives to include your cancer treatment.

Frustration can also arise from your own wish to be physically strong, while knowing that this is not possible all the time. This can be hard for your family and friends too – you may feel that people are walking on eggshells around you, trying not to offend you by treating you as an invalid while at the same time making sure you have all the support you need. It is a difficult balance to strike, and there will inevitably be times when you or other people make the wrong judgement. There will be moments when you will feel like shouting, 'Why doesn't someone help me?' or at the other end of the scale, 'I really don't need your help with this.' Similarly, those around you will be wondering whether an offer of help will be welcomed or considered an insult. The only way to find out is to keep all the lines of communication open and to be as flexible as you can. It will take time to reach the right balance – and just to make matters more complicated, the balance may change, from day to day or week to week or gradually over time.

It will be tough for your close family to adjust too, however supportive they are. While they will be doing their utmost to help you practically and emotionally, those who are closest to you will also be going through a period of shock and fear for the future. If you have previously taken pride in your emotional strength and ability to support others, remaining calm and strong at times of crisis, you may feel that it is incumbent upon you to do so now. And yet you may feel unable to, and need to draw on the support of others. Your family will not look to you to be the 'strong' party, but it can be difficult to shake off old habits. This can lead to a sense of emotional confusion for all concerned, and you will all need to allow time for relationships to reach a new balance.

This will have different effects for different people, some practical and some emotional. For example, there may be certain tasks which you have always carried out but which you are not capable of at the moment. Handing over responsibility for these can feel like a failure on your part, and might initially cause some upheaval as your family or friends adjust their own routines to accommodate you. It is sometimes more difficult to be the recipient than the giver of help, and you may find it hard to sit on the sidelines and take a less active role, especially if people don't do things 'your' way.

After my first four-week stay in hospital, it was wonderful to be home but difficult at first to accept that I had had no part in tying up the loose ends following the sale of our business nor in dealing with any domestic matters which had cropped up. Helen had been keeping me up to date with what was happening, but had obviously had to take complete control, make decisions and deal with things on a day-to-day basis herself. I would probably have done things no differently, but needed to quibble at times just to feel that I still had an opinion which mattered! My parents too had been very supportive in helping us sort out practical issues at home, and I'm sure I was less than gracious at times in accepting their help simply because it was so hard to accept that we needed it. I desperately needed to feel part of all that was going on around me and to assert my independence in some way – it was as

89

if after being in a relatively helpless state as a 'patient' for so long, I needed to regain my status as a functioning human being with a brain.

It is not easy to be a spectator while other people continue with their lives, and this can emphasize your situation painfully. Allow time and keep talking – relationships do reach a new state of equilibrium.

Changes in image

Both our self-image and the way we are perceived by others are built up over years and develop gradually. A cancer diagnosis can have a damaging effect on how you perceive yourself and affect how well you cope with your cancer. There will be times when you feel isolated from the world around you, as if you are not playing the role you want. You might fear that others will perceive you as weak or helpless, unable to manage for yourself, even if you had previously viewed yourself as a strong and independent person.

In fact, this fear is more likely to be imagined than real. Of course your family and friends will be sympathetic about your cancer and want to do all they can to help you. But this does not mean that they perceive you purely as a cancer patient, and no longer as their husband/son/brother/friend, etc. You will almost certainly feel that you have 'changed' as a person as a result of your cancer, in terms of your outlook or changed perspective on life. This is not the same as becoming a lesser person!

Keeping in touch is one of the best ways to guard against losing your confidence and sense of self. Your cancer will necessarily be on your mind for a large proportion of your time, either because you are thinking about it or because it has practical implications for your deeds and actions. This can increase your sense of isolation. Try to ensure that your family and friends keep you informed about what is happening in their lives, so that you continue to feel involved. Seemingly trivial details about what A said to B or how your friend's new job is progressing are valuable for keeping you in touch and ensuring that you continue to have the same conversations you always had rather than talking always about your cancer. Of course, you will talk about your cancer too – it is part of your life – but a balance can be struck so that you do not become shut off in a restricted world of your own.

Counselling and support

However well you cope and however strong your support network, there may be periods when you feel that extra help in the form of professional counselling would be valuable. You might find it hard to accept that you can't manage on your own with the support of your family and friends, and this is often a stumbling block to seeking counselling. Feeling a need to talk to someone outside your family and circle of friends is not a sign of weakness, and you might find that discussing your cancer and how it has affected you with a professional with whom you have no emotional ties helps you to express yourself differently.

It is important that you and your family know where to find counselling when you need it. While you are in hospital as an in-patient, your medical team will be able to advise you of support provided in the hospital. Some hospitals also provide ongoing counselling sessions for cancer patients once they have returned home, whereby you can return to the hospital for, say, weekly counselling. Alternatively, your GP should be able to advise you about the type and availability of counsellors in your area. Do try asking your doctors first, as they should be informed about the type of services available both in your locality and for your particular circumstances.

If you prefer, there are also organizations which you can contact for help and advice. For their telephone numbers and addresses see the 'Useful contacts' section at the end of the book.

The Help for Health Trust provides free, confidential health information (not specific medical advice), including details of self-help and support groups and a leaflet library. The Cancer Information Service is run by specially trained cancer nurses who answer queries by phone about all aspects of living with cancer. The Cancer Counselling Service has professional counsellors who are available to talk through the problems which can arise from living with cancer.

These are a few examples of national services, and by checking in leaflets at your hospital or at your local Cancer Information Centre you may find local specialist services or support groups as well.

Some people find that joining a support group is valuable for meeting other patients in similar circumstances away from a hospital setting. Support groups are split both by location and type of cancer. Some exist for the benefit of all cancer patients in a local area, while others are targeted at patients with specific cancers. Again, your hospital or GP or a national organization such as BACUP (British Association of Cancer United Patients) will be able to help to find a support group in your area. CancerLink publishes an annual *Directory of Cancer Support and Self Help*, a national publication containing details of several hundred cancer support groups and their activities. It is free to people with cancer. If no support group exists in your area, you might feel motivated to establish one.

What can a support group offer you? Some are called 'self-help' groups and this sums up their *raison d'être* – they exist for people sharing a common experience, so that they can pool thoughts and resources with others who understand first-hand how it feels to live with cancer. A support group can supply information and advice, as well as providing a forum for discussion of individual experiences or for airing grievances or negative feelings which you find too difficult to express to your family.

Simply being part of a group can boost your sense of control and make you feel stronger – we often feel that there is strength in numbers. Meeting other people who have experienced similar feelings and difficulties and who really understand what you are going through can help you to feel less isolated. You might even find that although you join a group seeking support for yourself, you are also able to give something back – by listening, or providing a snippet of information, or passing on your personal ways of coping. The sense that you are able to contribute something positive from an essentially negative experience can feel very satisfying.

Talking about life and death

One of the first questions in the mind of every newly diagnosed cancer patient is 'How long have I got?' Whether or not you voice the question and however good your likely prognosis, it is an issue which will not go away. Even now when some cancers can be treated very effectively we tend to associate the word 'cancer' with impending death. When you are experiencing the initial shock of diagnosis, it is very difficult to take seriously a doctor's view that treatment can be potentially curative or that a substantial period of remission might be achieved. From a patient's point of view, a preoccupation with dying is partly a reaction to the shock of diagnosis and partly a tendency to think the very worst so that any future news can't be any worse. It is as if in the early stages, we need to harden ourselves to bad news.

A fear of death is natural and inevitable, whatever your circumstances. Part of the process of coming to terms with your diagnosis is the fear that cancer is potentially a life-threatening disease, and that you are the person under threat. This is not at all the same as saying that all men with cancer have only a short remaining life span. It is rather that the experience of shock, disbelief and negative feelings is one of the stages of adapting to life with cancer.

As a society we shy away from talking about death, to the extent that it is regarded as a taboo subject. We use euphemisms such as 'passing on' to soften our words, rather than the harsher and final-sounding 'died'. Discussing death is difficult and you may struggle to find the right words to express how you feel, wanting to acknowledge the seriousness of cancer yet avoiding brutal and harsh words: 'This looks very serious and I'm frightened about the future' or 'I'm afraid the future is not looking too bright for me at the moment'. Your family and friends will find it a difficult subject to approach too, and you may find that some are unwilling or unable to discuss it. Responses like, 'But you're looking so much better, you'll be well in no time' or simply 'Don't talk like that' can feel like a rejection of your need to talk about *your* fears. This is not a reflection on you, but an indication of other people's inability (because of their own fear) to put your feelings before their own.

If you are willing to talk about fears for your prognosis, you may find that sympathetic family members and friends are relieved to have the opportunity to confide in you their own worries about your future, their fears of losing you and what that would mean to them. This can bring about some very emotional exchanges, but they can also bring huge relief that the subject is 'permitted' and that they can say what they really feel.

At times your feelings may become overwhelming and it is very important to have an outlet for them. If you do not feel able to talk to your close family or friends, then do try to speak with your doctors or nurses. They will be happy to spend time with you or to arrange for you to speak with a counsellor. Bottling up emotions on such a traumatic subject will not help you, either emotionally or in your efforts to maintain physical strength.

Things you can do

Confronting the concept of dying is a separate process to confronting the reality of your cancer. If your doctor has told you that your prognosis is not good or has worsened, then you will need to come to terms with that fact in the way that is best for you and your loved ones. It is very hard to accept, let alone to come to terms with, and it can be tempting to refuse to face it by choosing not to talk about it, even though it may be constantly on your mind. If you are continuing to have treatment, then hope for a 'miracle cure' can easily remain stronger in your mind than the likely reality that you are not going to recover – it is a kind of coping mechanism.

It is rare for a person to completely refuse to acknowledge approaching death, when this becomes inevitable – although it can be complicated by the fact that so many variables are in play that no doctor can predict how long a patient will live. Most people do reach some form of acceptance, although this does not necessarily entail frequent and long discussion of the process. You may be inclined not to talk about it and try to put it out of your mind. On the other hand, you might be the sort of person for whom some discussion is important. Some people choose to go a stage further, and express their wishes and feelings about dying in a Living Will. This is a document which expresses your wishes for your medical and nursing care as you approach death. It may be that this is not strictly necessary in the sense that you know you will be well cared for. It can nevertheless help by giving a sense of control over your treatment right up to your death and help your family by allowing them to be sure that they are doing just as you would wish.

When Neil's prognosis suddenly worsened considerably, we prepared three documents together:

- a Living Will which set out his wishes regarding his medical care;
- a 'Death Plan' which expressed his wishes on more general

matters such as whether he would like to continue having visitors as his death approached, the music he would like played and other issues which impinged on the environment and atmosphere in which he died;

- Advance Funeral Wishes which set out detailed instructions for his funeral and burial.

This was an emotional but in some ways comforting exercise. Once the documents were prepared (and after we had sorted out other practicalities) we felt freer to concentrate our energies on Neil's continuing treatment and our time together in the knowledge that these logistical issues were taken care of. It also allowed Neil the reassurance that he had expressed his wishes and that even if he became unable to communicate his thoughts adequately, they would be adhered to – which, of course, they were. The knowledge that we had discussed these incredibly important issues together was tremendously helpful to me, as I could feel at each stage that I was 'doing the right thing' – vital both at the time and in retrospect.

A good source of further information and pro-forma documents which you can tailor to your own needs is *The New Natural Death Handbook* produced by The Natural Death Centre. The Centre also produces a set of forms which includes a Living Will. The book *What You Really Need to Know About Cancer* by Dr Robert Buckman also includes a useful pro-forma Living Will, with additional clauses covering, for example, legal liability.

Some people make a Living Will while in perfectly good health to cover unforeseen eventualities such as severe and lasting brain damage or an advanced degenerative disease. The point of a Living Will is to make specific statements about the type of care and medical intervention you wish to receive and, equally important, not to receive, if you are close to dying in case it becomes difficult or impossible to make decisions yourself. If you have cancer and are not expected to recover, the circumstances are more specific, and your Living Will can reflect this. There has been much ethical debate about patients' 'refusal' of treatment (although this is not necessarily what a Living Will expresses), and it is important that you talk about your Living Will to your GP and the doctors treating you to ensure that they accept and will act in accordance with your wishes. In practice, your wishes are likely to reflect the treatment you would in any case have received, but your sense of control will be enhanced if you make these statements yourself.

It is a good idea to use a pro-forma for your Living Will, and adapt it as necessary – although there is nothing to stop you drafting your own version. Please bear in mind that the points mentioned below do not cover all circumstances or illnesses and are purely an outline of some of the issues you might wish to consider, such as:

- your views on medical intervention such as blood transfusions, artificial ventilation or antibiotics;
- whether you wish distressing symptoms to be controlled by medications such as painkillers, even though these may shorten life;
- your views about physical comfort, and artificial feeding and hydration (as opposed simply to maintaining comfort by having mouth and lips moistened);
- whether you wish to die at home, if this is possible, or at the hospital where you have been treated or at a hospice;
- any care you specifically refuse, such as transfer to a 'high tech' intensive care facility;
- who is to be responsible for taking decisions on your behalf, should this be necessary (wife/partner/parent/son/daughter, etc).

A Death Plan (also available as a pro-forma from The Natural Death Centre) covers more general points such as:

- (reiterate) where you prefer to be cared for;
- the name of your next of kin and whether you have made a Living Will;
- whether you would like to continue having visitors when close to death;
- whether you wish it made clear to visitors that you are dying;
- if you would like your wife/partner to sleep in the same bed/room as you;
- any loved ones you would particularly like to be involved in your care;
- your religious/spiritual philosophy (if any) and how this is to be applied to your dying;
- the 'ministrations' you might appreciate – music, hand held, prayers, massage, reading, etc;

- who you would like with you at the moment of your death;
- (reiterate) feelings about pain control.

There may be other specific points you wish to include – the document is an expression of *your* personal wishes.

Your Living Will and Death Plan should be signed and witnessed, and copies given to those responsible for your care (GP, hospital doctor, hospice doctor, etc).

During Neil's last days, I felt thankful that he had wanted to make his views and wishes clear. Through the sense of unreality it gave us something to focus on, to ensure that the music he requested was playing, that the comforts he requested were available, the people he wanted close were there. As he gradually became less conscious, I consulted both his Living Will and Death Plan several more times, to make sure I had missed nothing. The hospice staff were also hugely obliging, and made sure they too were familiar with their contents, volunteering the loan of a portable CD player, for example, so that we could play music easily. It made a big difference not to be constantly wondering whether we were doing as Neil would have wanted – because he had told us.

7

Coping with daily life

There is no 'right' way to live with cancer. It would be so much easier if doctors could not only prescribe treatments and drugs, but also ways to manage best and to cope with each new situation. Unfortunately, life is rarely that clear-cut and living with cancer certainly isn't! You will need time to adjust but with some will-power and determination and the help of your family and friends, 'normal' life need not come to a standstill.

There are many factors which will affect how you manage from day to day, and no two men will feel exactly the same even in very similar circumstances. Your symptoms and the effects of your treatment may not interfere too much with your daily life if your cancer was detected early. If it was more advanced and had already taken some toll on your body before treatment, convalescence could take longer and the impact on your daily life will be greater. Similarly, the physical effects of your cancer and treatment may hit you less hard if you are basically a strong and fit person than someone in less good general health. What is important is to take notice of what your body is telling you and not to fight it.

The day of my first consultation with an oncologist will be remembered as the Day of the Corridors! We had arrived at the general hospital and their once-weekly cancer clinic, and I was feeling weak and terrible. I am convinced that all hospitals have a cunning plan which ensures that all patients and their carers should walk all possible corridors before they arrive at their chosen destination. In a large, sprawling hospital such a trek really can feel like a marathon. The best way to counter this – which did not occur to us until we staggered out post-consultation and after another trek to the X-ray department, of course – is either to hijack the first spare wheelchair you come across (look in the lobbies around the entrance to any hospital or ask at reception), or if this is impractical insist on the help of a porter to help you navigate those long corridors. Do remember that you might have only a limited amount of energy and using it up in non-productive ways is not a constructive use of a scarce resource!

If you are the sort of person who would rather crawl into work with a burning temperature and a raging headache rather than admit that the 'flu has got the better of you, then listening to your body *and* acting on it may take some effort. You might be tempted to understate your symptoms or side-effects, both to others in an attempt to prevent people treating you purely as a 'cancer patient' and to yourself so that you feel able to continue with your 'normal' life. A balancing act is needed here – of course it is helpful to lead as normal a life as possible rather than withdrawing completely and immersing yourself in your cancer. On the other hand, you need to be aware of your limitations and to modify your daily routines accordingly. This will require a good deal of trial and error, and you will misjudge your physical strength at times.

It will help too if you don't test your body by pushing it to its physical limits. Especially coming home after a stay in hospital, it is easy to overstretch yourself even if you have been told to 'take it easy'. Simple tasks around the house might take more energy and conscious effort than usual – you wouldn't usually think twice about making a cup of tea, but this may leave you needing a rest afterwards. On some days you will feel stronger than others, and can take pleasure in tasks or hobbies which are too much for you on other days. The days when you have no energy can be intensely frustrating, but you won't gain anything if you fight it! This does not mean you should never try to be active and just sit in a chair or retire to bed and do nothing. Don't give up, but try to accept that for a while at least, you need to conserve your energy and use it carefully. Only you can judge your limits, and you mustn't be too proud to impose them on yourself and others. It is crazy knowingly to exhaust yourself just to prove a point, for example, preparing your own lunch when someone has offered to do it for you. What exactly do you succeed in proving? And to whom?

If you have always worked and led an active life, it can be tough to accept that now there are times when you haven't the physical strength to do so. Whatever the pace of your life up to now, be it frenetic and dictated by heavy pressures of work and family or more gentle, you will have to slow down. Admitting this is often the most difficult step to take, as if there is some shame associated with a loss of physical strength. Nobody will think any worse of you if you aren't able to go to work every day, or indeed, if you need to take longer periods of sick leave. No one will laugh at you or condemn you or stop considering you a friend if you can't play football at weekends or go to the pub or entertain until the small hours.

It is still natural to want to preserve as much normality as possible in your life. After the shock of a cancer diagnosis, you can gain reassurance from familiar routines, and they can provide some stability in a period of shock and stress. The people around you can probably make the greatest difference to how you feel, but you will need to feel that you are not entirely dependent on them and can also help yourself. Being assigned the status of a 'patient' can knock your self-confidence and it is important to feel that you can preserve some independence and the sense of self which you achieve from structuring your own life and deciding for yourself what you do and when.

Again, there will be times when you are treading a fine line. On some days you may be able to go to work or visit a friend or be active at home. There will be other times when it is a struggle to drag yourself out of bed and you feel exhausted after brushing your teeth in the morning. On your 'tired' days, you may want to do nothing but rest – even conversation may be too much. Accept this, even if you do feel wretched that you are so powerless. Use your 'good' days to best advantage, so that you can regain some sense of control in your life. For example, decide on something you would like to achieve that day. It doesn't matter how small it is – writing a letter, making a phone call, walking down the garden – or if you are feeling good, going out for a short walk, visiting a friend or asking someone to drive you to a favourite place. Don't set yourself tasks which you know you are unlikely to manage – there is no point in setting yourself up for a sense of failure. It is surprising how a small achievement can contribute to a more positive frame of mind. Don't expect too much from yourself – treat yourself gently.

There will be times when practical help is very welcome. It may be hard to admit that you cannot be completely independent, but it is foolish to refuse help purely on the grounds of bloody-mindedness! If you are recovering from surgery, or feeling tired as a result of radiotherapy or at a low point in your chemotherapy cycle, you can feel physically very drained and weak. It makes sense to conserve your energy for yourself, and take up people's offers to cook you a meal, drive you to the hospital, walk the dog, do some shopping, cut the grass – the list goes on. Help from family or friends with seemingly small tasks can make a big difference to the quality of your life, allowing you to use your energy to take pleasure in the company of friends or to carry out the tasks you want, rather than need, to.

When people ask, 'Is there anything I can do?', they mean their offer to be taken seriously. Even if you do not need help at that time, you can still say 'I'm fine at the moment, but maybe I could ask you later when I'm not feeling so good.' You could also check whether they would be prepared to help with specific tasks – 'Would you mind driving me to the bank/supermarket/post office when you next go to town?'; or asking if they would be happy just to spend some time with you: 'I know you're busy now, but perhaps at the weekend you could come and visit for an hour?' It is sometimes easier for everyone if some basic 'guidelines' for visitors are worked out and if your family and friends have some idea of the type of help you would welcome and what you would prefer to deal with yourself. This will also help you in maintaining a sense of control over your daily life, rather than allowing others to decide what is 'best' for you.

Work

If you have a job, you need to think carefully about whether you can continue to work. It may be that the decision is clear-cut and you know that you will be out of action for a period of weeks or months. In many cases though, it is impossible to predict in advance how you will react to your treatment, however well-informed you are about its side-effects. You might find that you can work part-time, perhaps a few days each week or a few hours each day. You may feel perfectly well and strong enough to work one day and exhausted the next.

It is sensible to start by asking your doctor's opinion about whether you are fit to work. Although it is difficult in many circumstances for a doctor to give a definitive answer, their advice will be useful when you discuss the issue with your employer. You may be advised to ease yourself back to work gently and to ensure you take sick leave if you are feeling low, or to start by working part-time. Alternatively, your doctor may advise you to stop working until your treatment is completed or until you are physically stronger.

The next step is to talk to your employer to make sure no misunderstandings arise about whether or not you will be at work (or ask somebody to talk to your employer on your behalf). You may be unable to guarantee from day to day when you can work, and it is important that this is fully understood. It is even more important that you are not in a state of worry about work commitments – you need your energy for yourself.

For those fortunate to be in some form of paid work, perhaps the most critical decision is exactly what to do with this activity which has previously, probably, dominated your waking existence. The decision will vary dramatically between individuals – employed, self-employed, attitude of employer, full-time, part-time, etc – but for me the key decision was surprisingly easy. We were running a chartered accountancy practice which I had established some seven years earlier and there was never any doubt in either of our minds that we both had to stop working and use all energies available on the cancer. I think we both knew that this would, of course, make us much poorer – although I am not certain we then realized the full extent and link between illness and poverty – but that there was absolutely no alternative.

I was so, so lucky in one key aspect. I had formed a wonderful friendship and mutual professional support with a friend who ran a similar practice in Devon. Without a second thought, he came to see us and worked flat out for a fortnight to sell the business as quickly and profitably as possible. The end result was that within a fortnight of C-day and with the truly heroic efforts of my friend (and his wife 'holding the fort' at home) and the goodwill and integrity of the purchaser, the business was sold and we faced a future with a dramatically reduced income! Except that we had the time to deal with the cancer.

I know that this situation will only apply precisely to a very limited number of people, and that the level of horsetrading between employee and employer and the trade-off between income and time will be much more complex for most. All I would stress is that for us it was a great liberation to be free of the tyranny of time and resources which our work ate up. All efforts had to go into facing the cancer.

102

If you do decide or have to give up work, even for a relatively short time, you will obviously need to consider the financial implications. Money – or a lack of it – is one of the most common sources of stress. Anxieties about how to pay the mortgage next month or where the money for the electricity bill or the children's school uniforms is coming from are the last thing you need – but at the same time are issues which can't be avoided. If you do not have any other source of income, you need advice at an early stage about any benefits you are entitled to claim and whether you will be able to manage. These benefits are covered in more detail in Chapter 8. You may also feel great bitterness that your cancer has forced you into this position and created yet further problems. Your family might find this hard to accept too, resenting the situation while not wanting to add to your worries. Do get advice if you need it – a social worker will be available at your hospital who has experience of these issues. He or she can guide you through the system and save you time and energy.

For many of us, work occupies a significant proportion of our waking hours and an important position in our lives. It often dominates almost to the extent of defining who we are – when we are introduced to someone, one of the first topics of conversation is frequently, 'Do you work?' or 'What do you do for a living?' Even though you will be preoccupied with your cancer and treatment, giving up work can leave a void in your life. If you are at home, you will need to find ways of staving off the inevitable boredom, and making sure you don't miss out on the social contact which work naturally provides. If it is physically possible, you might prefer to continue working at a reduced level to preserve some sense of normality in your life. Different people have different priorities and you, in consultation with your doctors, will need to decide what is right for you.

One man in his 30s being treated for stomach cancer who was employed by a bank continued to work whenever he could throughout his chemotherapy, with prearranged time off for his hospital treatment every three weeks. He felt that this would prevent him from 'climbing the walls' at home. He wasn't always well enough to go to work, but preferred to do so whenever possible. Another in similar circumstances felt he needed to give up work for the duration of his treatment and convalescence, in order to concentrate solely on fighting his cancer. The decision might be made for you by your state of health or the nature of your job, but if not, try to decide what is best for you and *not* what other people expect of you.

If much of your life has revolved around work, it can be hard to conceive of such a dramatic change to your routine, let alone to admit that you are not always physically able to manage your job. In telling your employer and colleagues, you may fear that their perception of your capabilities will be affected or that they may not be entirely sympathetic about your cancer. Perhaps you feel determined to continue working at all costs, simply to prove that you can, or feel that you must from a sense of insecurity about your career prospects in the future.

The best policy is honesty with your employer. If your doctors have advised you that you will need time off for treatment, either occasional days or more prolonged periods, don't imply that you will not need any sick leave. If your case is less clear-cut and you may need odd days off, make this clear. It will be easier for you and your colleagues to plan around your likely absences if you are explicit with them about what to expect. How you and they will cope with this will depend very much on the nature of your work. Maybe a colleague can cover for you on an ad hoc basis when necessary. If your work doesn't allow for that, some careful forward planning of your workload will be needed, which will require you to be as open with your colleagues as possible. There is usually a means of resolving this, either by using temporary staff, delegating elsewhere or reallocating some of your work. Losing touch and getting left behind might be a fear – but perhaps you can arrange with colleagues to keep you up-to-date if you are absent for any length of time.

When you are not fully fit, even a job which is not physically demanding can leave you exhausted at the end of the day. Frustrating though it may be, this is a time when you must put yourself first and not the demands (or perceived demands) of your job. If you insist on working against medical advice or your better judgement just to prove that you can, you will find it even harder to maintain your physical strength – and you need it for yourself above all else.

Daily life

Whatever your circumstances and whether or not you have a job, your 'normal' life will be disrupted to a greater or lesser extent by your cancer. You might want to behave as if nothing has changed, but the harsh fact still remains that you are living with cancer. However effectively you cope with it, it will impose limitations on you. People who know about it will treat you differently, probably unconsciously. It takes time to get used to these changes, to try not to be angry about them and to learn to be flexible and adapt your life where necessary.

Frustration

It is tempting to try to do too much at first, to test the boundaries of your strength. You may feel fine and full of energy for days or weeks on end, then gradually find that the cumulative effects of radiotherapy or chemotherapy are taking their toll and sapping your energy. Many people who have lived through cancer say that mind-numbing tiredness is one of the most difficult side-effects to bear. Feeling exhausted after making the effort to get out of bed is not very conducive to a positive frame of mind and a fighting spirit! Long-term tiredness (or even short-term tiredness) can lead to intense frustration at your own helplessness. When some well-meaning soul advises you for the umpteenth time to 'Try to relax and get some rest' you may feel like screaming (if you have the energy), 'What do you think I am trying to do? Run a marathon?'

Using your time

You will need to find ways to hold on to your sanity when your usual activities are severely curtailed. An understanding listener can make a big difference when you need to express your frustrations, but you still need to find ways to pass the time and occupy your mind. Television or videos or radio might keep you entertained at first, but these can wear thin and you may start to feel too passive, as if you need more stimulation than a TV picture. What you need to find are pastimes which you enjoy but which are not too strenuous, which stave off frustration but which you can put aside immediately if you need to rest. The most simple pastimes can often be the most effective.

Reading is fine if you enjoy it and can concentrate. Books and glossy magazines tend to be expensive, but you can ask a friend or relative to visit the local libraries and charity shops as a cheaper alternative. If friends ask if they can bring you anything when they visit, a magazine might be a suitable present. If you find it difficult to concentrate or simply find it hard work to hold a book for long periods, you could try listening to books on tape, which are widely available at libraries. As well as books, a whole variety of television and radio programmes can be obtained on tape. If you don't already own one, a personal stereo might be an extremely useful gift.

Listening to music can be therapeutic as well as pleasurable. Choose your music to suit your mood – sometimes loud, 'angry' music can provide a better release for your emotions than the more obvious calm and relaxing choices.

Writing letters, if you are able to, gives you the opportunity to keep people in touch with how you are and is sometimes an easier way of expressing your thoughts than a conversation. We are accustomed to using the phone rather than letters to maintain contact with family and friends, and you may feel, 'What's the point of writing when I can pick up the phone. Anyway, I haven't written a personal letter since I was at school.' It may take you a while to get started, but there's a sense of satisfaction gained with signing off a letter. We all love to receive a personal letter, and you may find that people's pleasure in hearing from you gives you a boost too.

Taking the theme of putting your thoughts on paper a step further, keeping a diary or journal of your experiences and thoughts during your treatment can provide another outlet for your emotions. It doesn't have to be anything grand – perhaps a notebook in which you record notes of how your treatment is progressing, how you are feeling, the positive and negative sides of your experience.

Games are a good source of distraction and can help to keep your mind ticking over. Those which are not too long, intricate and involved are generally preferable, such as card games, backgammon or Scrabble. If your concentration levels are not brilliant or you have a tendency to become tired, these can be quickly started and easily put aside or picked up later.

Sometimes it's useful to have an ongoing 'project' to give you a sense of purpose and to provide another thread of continuity in your life at a time of disruption. Try not to choose anything which will require constant physical effort, but ideally a project which can be picked up and put down whenever you wish. It might be something you had always promised yourself you would do 'when you had the time', or something completely new or something you have been meaning to return to for years. It will obviously depend on your particular interests as well as your physical capabilities: keeping a diary of your experience of cancer, cataloguing your record or CD collection, learning a new computer program, taking up sketching again, helping in some way with a cancer support group. . . . As well as helping you to feel that you are able to use your time resourcefully, you will have something tangible as an end result.

Alternatively, you might choose to plan forward for a project to be undertaken when your treatment is over – something constructive to look forward to. This could be connected with your house (plans for your garden or decorating); associated with work (the outline for an idea or project you have always wanted to develop but never had the time); or something entirely personal (choosing the destination for the holiday you plan to take after your treatment).

If you have (or if someone can arrange) access to one, a portable PC can open up new horizons. Whether you are accustomed to more sophisticated technology or have always been a technophobe, you can use it as a word processor, to play games or for whichever programs suit your needs and interests.

'Treats' can give you a boost too, even if they do suggest childhood. What they are depends entirely upon you; the point is that they represent something which is a luxury for you, even if a very small one. This might be something to eat or drink, a CD or record, a book or magazine, a game or gadget, an item of clothing. . . . It doesn't need to cost much, but should make you feel good. Have regular treats – they are good for you! Make sure other people know about them, but don't let them embarrass you by spending large sums of money or going to great trouble.

If you are well enough, avoiding being confined to home can make a difference to your state of mind. You may be content to spend more time than usual quietly at home, but gazing at the same four walls can leave you feeling stir-crazy after a relatively short time. Going out can also boost your self-assurance. If your mobility is not particularly affected, then this may be easy for you. If on the other hand, trips or visits need to be planned and depend on how you feel on a given day, then they can assume a greater significance. You might visit friends, or favourite old haunts or new places further afield. The location and purpose is less important than dispelling the sense that your life revolves entirely around your cancer. You do need other distractions in your mind, and 'a change of scenery' can help. Similarly, taking a holiday either during or after your treatment can provide a boost: even a break of a few days away can be very beneficial.

Having always led such a busy life, the enforced inaction of the first six weeks or so following my diagnosis were an alien concept to me – but at the time I was too ill to have any choice. After that initial period, I actually found to my surprise that I was enjoying having this 'leisure' time (although not the reason it was forced upon me!) and for the first time in years, I had time to call my own. It was also a period for reflection and reassessment of my priorities, but quite apart from that, I enjoyed being able to sit in the garden and read or write letters, have friends to visit, spend days on end at local cricket matches, go to my favourite record shops (going unaccompanied for the first time was a big day!), and spend time pottering around the countryside, going to places we'd always promised we'd visit 'when we had the time'. Our finances were pretty stretched, but our lifestyle was not exactly extravagant at that time and our pleasures were generally simple ones. We saw this as a finite period, which would change again when my treatment was complete, so we thought we might as well make the most of it.

It is not only at home you will need ways to fill your time, but also in hospital if you are being treated as an in-patient. The same principles apply, although your days will be punctuated by your treatment, by drug rounds, ward rounds, mealtimes and so on. Even if the environment is busy and bustling and you have family and friends to pay regular visits, time can drag simply because you want to have your treatment as quickly as possible and get home again.

By my third or fourth chemotherapy cycle I was feeling much stronger and fitter and more like my 'old' self, and found I had to switch into what we called 'hospital mode' as soon as we walked through the hospital entrance. As an impatient person who likes to get on with things, I found the waiting around and the inevitable delays incredibly frustrating at first – it seemed they were occurring just to annoy me. This, of course, is not the case – blood tests had to be taken and the results checked, chemo had to be ordered, I had to wait for a doctor to be available to examine me, drugs had to be ordered from the pharmacy, sometimes scans had to be organized. All of these procedures take time. 'Hospital mode' involved switching off the active part of my brain, turning on the TV or radio or settling down with a good book and trying to be the patient person I definitely am not – but there's no point in trying to fight the system. In fact, my three or four days often passed very quickly – but it didn't always feel that way, and the only solution for me was to switch off completely.

You and your family

Depending on the nature and extent of your cancer and treatment, living with cancer can have a dramatic effect on your family life. You may be less active and therefore less able to participate in your usual family routines, and your wife or partner may feel the strain of trying to cope both emotionally and practically. It will take time for children to adjust too and to understand that you can't always join in with their activities.

The extent of the effect on your family will obviously depend on how well or unwell you are. For example, if you need someone to be with you more or less constantly (not necessarily because you need constant 'nursing' care, but rather in case you need extra help at times during the day or night), then you need to work out ways of managing that. Your family might be able to manage this with occasional help from friends and relatives, but if you feel you need more support, your hospital or GP can put you in touch with organizations such as Marie Curie Cancer Care or Macmillan nurses, which can organize extra care at home. There is no charge to a patient or their family for this specialist nursing care (although many people feel motivated to support their work by means of a charitable donation).

The best ways of coping tend to evolve over time. You all need to be flexible, and to accept that while you want to preserve as much normality as possible, there will be times when plans go awry. Perhaps a planned day out can't go ahead because you feel too unwell, causing disappointment to your children. You may feel frustrated and even guilty that your cancer is such a dominant factor in your lives. It *is* hard, and the desire to avoid disappointing others is strong, but looking after yourself has to remain your top priority.

Physical activity and exercise

However strong you are, your treatment will affect your physical well-being. You may lose weight or suffer nausea or increasing lethargy, as well as experiencing side-effects specific to your treatment. You might wake in the morning feeling strong and well and unwittingly overtax yourself within a few hours. The idea of resting for the remainder of the day can be intensely frustrating. You may not *want* to sit quietly and watch the television or read the newspapers! Enforced physical inaction is a tangible and constant reminder of your cancer but, however irritating, only you can dictate the right pace of life for you.

For example, many courses of chemotherapy are given on a three-weekly cycle. You may discover with experience that there are points in the cycle when you feel the side-effects of the drugs most keenly, are particularly low, have very little energy and little desire for visitors or activity. At another point in the cycle, you may feel much stronger and want to be more active. Your medical team will advise you if you are likely to have low points in your cycle, but the effects of chemotherapy do vary from person to person. In the first cycle, however much information you are given beforehand, you won't know from personal experience how you will be affected. Thereafter, your personal experience will be valuable in guiding your day-to-day life. For example, if you know you feel low on days 7 to 10 after your chemotherapy, you can plan ahead and take life very gently on those days. Keeping some form of diary may be useful, even if you just make a brief note each day of how you feel: 'Day 15 – felt strong, went to work today' or 'Day 9 – nausea bad, couldn't eat, slept badly'.

Judging the level of physical exercise or activity that is right for you may be tricky as your physical energy goes through unpredictable periods of improvement and decline. If you are well enough, it is good to exercise in some form if you can, but as gently as necessary – if a very short walk is enough, then don't push yourself further. You are not trying to prove anything to anyone!

Ask your doctor's guidance about your physical limitations and try to respect that advice. Your doctor will not be able to tell you exactly what you can and cannot do, but you may have questions about whether you can, for example, go swimming or play a round of golf or go to the gym. Your doctor should be able to advise you about any activities which should be avoided or approached with caution, or indeed, any which would be especially beneficial.

You might be eager to become more physically active again or you might be surprised by psychological hurdles which have to be crossed first. If an operation has caused some physical change or what you perceive to be a disfigurement, however minor, then this can change your attitude about your body and make you feel uncertain either about your physical capabilities or your willingness to have your body 'on show'. If the prospect of undressing in the open changing room at the gym or swimming pool leaves you feeling very uncomfortable, then don't force yourself into that particular activity. It is worth reiterating that there is no 'right' way to approach this – you must follow your instincts.

Companionship

We all enjoy spending time with friends and loved ones, and in any case, the stimulation of visitors can be beneficial. There will be times when you feel the need for almost constant support and companionship. If you are experiencing a 'low' period and feel anxious and vulnerable then the company of a loved one or a good friend is invaluable – how often do we admit in times of stress or crisis (although usually after the event) that 'I couldn't have got through it without X'? At other times you may prefer to be alone with your own thoughts or to go out on your own in order to feel more independent. Your needs will vary, and while it may not be possible for family and friends always to be with you when you need them, it is helpful if they can understand when and why you need them most.

If you live alone or your wife/partner works full-time, then you will need to devise ways to ensure you have sufficient company and support. Even if you are generally happy to be alone, it is important that you do not feel isolated and unable to ask for companionship when you need it. Picking up the phone and letting a friend or relative know that you'd appreciate a visit can be hard at first – there may be some sense of admission that you can't manage on your own, which you find difficult. This is not, of course, the case – often, people are delighted to be asked, and flattered that you have chosen them. It is very important not to let pride stand in your way! If you do usually live alone, it is likely that hospital staff will insist on arrangements to be made for your support and care before you are able to go home after treatments. This is not because they do not trust you to look after yourself, but because side-effects and problems can be unpredictable, and it is in nobody's interest not to take suitable precautions.

From a practical point of view, you may need more support than usual with everyday tasks which you have always undertaken without a second thought, such as preparing meals or getting around and out of the house. Treatment can have unexpected effects on your physical strength and stamina, and it is important to make sure that back-up is available when you need it. This doesn't necessarily mean you need someone to look after you full-time, although one option is to ask a relative or friend to stay with you for a time. If this is not feasible or desirable, your district nurse can arrange to visit you at home each day, and Marie Curie or Macmillan nurses can offer more specialist nursing care if you need it. Your GP can visit to check that you are coping with your medications and any side-effects. An occupational therapist can also advise on any special equipment to make managing at home easier for you.

Arrangements for both emotional and practical support may need to be more structured if you live or spend most of your time alone and can't rely on the presence of a wife or partner. You may have to make a more conscious effort to ensure that you have all the help you need – but this does not mean that you will manage any less effectively.

Relaxation

You may associate the concept of relaxation with classes full of women in leotards. This does not have to be the case! You will almost certainly undergo stresses which affect both your mind and body, and learning some basic relaxation techniques *can* help. This does not mean that you have to sit cross-legged on the floor chanting 'Om' – although if this suits you, then fine.

Simple breathing exercises in which you learn to breathe deeply and at a controlled rate can help to slow down your mind when your thoughts are racing. You can also incorporate simple physical exercises which help to relax your muscles, especially those in the neck and shoulders where many people carry much of their tension. You can ask your GP or at your hospital for help in learning these techniques. Some hospitals run classes and workshops, for exactly this purpose.

Using essential oils (aromatherapy) can have a pleasurable and calming effect. Oils can be used in the bath or diluted in a 'carrier' oil to use in massage (or simply rubbing into your hands or feet, for example) or to burn in an oil burner. Different oils have different properties and can help to promote relaxation – or simply be pleasant to use. Again, some of the nurses on your ward may have had training in the use of essential oils, or be able to recommend sources of information.

Some people use 'visualization techniques' – images of quiet or happy places, for example – to help them relax. Shutting your eyes and visualizing yourself in a favourite tranquil spot, imagining how you feel when you are there and allowing the image to take over your thoughts, if only for a minute or two, can have a calming effect.

If you want to practise relaxation techniques, you need to ensure you are in a quiet room without interruptions or excessive background noise. If you feel a little foolish at first, practise when you are alone. Remember that loved ones will be experiencing their own stresses too, and might like to share in practising your relaxation techniques.

For some people, relaxing may have a different meaning, such as the opportunity to watch a favourite TV programme or to listen to music undisturbed. What you do is less important than being aware of what makes you feel more relaxed and perhaps more refreshed afterwards. Achieving a more relaxed state may not directly affect your cancer treatment, but if it helps you to cope better in a calmer frame of mind, if only for a limited time, then it is surely worthwhile.

I had always been pretty sceptical about what I regarded as 'hippy stuff', although Helen swore by the physical and mental benefits of her yoga classes and the occasional massage. On the whole, I preferred to relax by listening to music, preferably very loudly and often joining in the lyrics myself, to the occasional alarm of our neighbours. I suffered some nerve damage in my hands and feet as a result of my chemotherapy, and Helen persuaded me that massaging them with essential oils might help to release some tension – and that I might just enjoy the sense of being pampered! This became a regular fixture – if my feet or hands were sore (or even if they weren't), she would rub them as gently or vigorously as felt comfortable while we were watching TV or chatting.

Although it could not directly help the nerve damage, it did help me to relax and she was right about the pampering!

Diet

Many people living with cancer do not experience problems eating or maintaining their weight, or suffer only temporary difficulties associated with their treatment. For some, though, eating and maintaining a reasonable diet becomes a serious and problematic issue. This might be a direct result of your cancer or of the side-effects of treatment. For example, nausea, a sore or dry mouth, changes in your sense of taste and sheer tiredness can all affect both your attitude to food and your ability and desire to eat.

A specialist dietician will be available at your hospital to advise about specific problems and solutions, and to recommend foods and drinks which might be more palatable, or nutritional supplements if necessary. Booklets are also available (such as *Diet and the Cancer Patient*, produced by BACUP) which contain guidance and ideas about boosting your diet if you are having difficulty eating. Similarly, if you have to follow a special diet, then you should receive help and advice on how best to go about it.

In spite of recognizing the importance of your diet, you may well become heartily fed up with other people's apparent obsession that you should eat the 'right things'. Plain tiredness may mean that you simply don't feel like preparing meals, or can't even be bothered to eat them, even though you know you should. However good your intentions to eat sensibly and well, this does not necessarily mean that you will take pleasure in your food. The act of preparing food can sometimes be off-putting too – certain smells might make you feel sick, or you may just find that having put together a meal with the best of intentions, you no longer fancy eating it.

It is important too to be allowed to eat the foods you find tempting (within reason!). You may feel completely put off certain foods you used to enjoy – highly spiced dishes like curries, for example, or dishes cooked in very rich sauces.

After a long initial stay in hospital when I couldn't eat, I found that above all I was craving 'comfort food'. The steroids I was taking to combat chemotherapy nausea had a dramatic effect on my appetite as well and Helen would sometimes find me in the kitchen ransacking the cupboards in search of tempting snacks!

Simple flavours were the best, with nothing too exotic or rich. Fish and chips was a favourite (I had dreamt obsessively in hospital about being able to eat fish and chips again), as were joints of roast meat and vegetables – uncomplicated flavours, but satisfying and filling – very important. My biggest disappointment was to find that beer was completely unpalatable!

Some people do find that their sense of taste is affected temporarily during chemotherapy, which can be disconcerting if you have been looking forward to a particular food only to find it tastes horrible. Trust to your instincts and eat the foods which tempt you. If you do have problems finding dishes to suit you, don't hesitate to contact the dietician at your hospital, who might be able to make suggestions – sometimes it can be hard to think laterally or imaginatively about food.

The ritual of eating is more complex than simply nourishing your body, and you may find mental barriers have to be overcome too. If you have lost some weight, you may be especially conscious of your body. Sitting down to meals with family and friends may also make you feel conscious that you are being watched and leave you feeling uncomfortable about not finishing a meal or wanting only a small amount. It *is* important to eat well, but it is also important for others to realize if this is difficult for you. Talking and letting people know your feelings will help – with your guidance and their support, problems will be resolved more easily.

If you live alone and need help with food and meals, then this should be organized by your GP or district nurse, and they will be able to organize extra support for you if you should need it.

Mobility

Mobility is important because it affects your sense of control and independence. Whatever your circumstances – whether you are in bed or using a wheelchair much of the time or simply not as energetic as usual – you need the right level of support to ensure a good level of comfort and the ability to do as much as you reasonably want to for yourself.

If you experience more difficulty than usual getting around the house you might consider making up a temporary 'bedroom' downstairs, as climbing stairs uses a lot of energy. If your bathroom is upstairs, then this may be less practical although you may be able to borrow equipment to solve this problem. The district nurse at your doctor's surgery will be able to advise you, perhaps in conjunction with an occupational therapist (who will know about specialist equipment or useful aids to make practical tasks easier for you).

There may be other equipment or small changes at home which would make a big difference to you. An adapted lavatory seat, a special cushion to sit on, the installation of handles to help you out of the bath, a new stair-rail or a walking frame to give you extra confidence are some examples. These may all be temporary measures, but can help you to feel less physically confined.

Experiencing reduced levels of energy is very common, and it will make a big difference if you are able – and willing – to rely on others more than usual. Getting up to fetch a book or make a cup of tea or prepare a snack may be more difficult than before, and although you may hate to feel like an 'invalid', it is often a relatively short-term problem. This does not mean that others will be constantly running around for you, nor that you should worry about 'being a burden' to them. Remember that you are undertaking this journey through your treatment together, and by working together you can vastly improve the quality of your life. Small measures can make a big difference.

Driving may be another activity you have always taken for granted. It is obviously foolish to drive if you are not fit to do so, and you also may need to consider the implications of any physical limitations caused by your cancer on your motor insurance. This may make no difference at all, but again, it would be foolish to be caught out.

If driving is not possible for you for a while, you may need to arrange for someone else to be available to drive you to your hospital appointments. Taxis or public transport may be a possibility for you, but you are likely to find that friends or family members are more than happy to save you the money or the time and trouble by driving you. Don't be afraid to ask! After all, you'd do the same for them.

8
Financial issues

Coping with your cancer is hard enough without added concern for your finances – which is a frequent source of stress and discord at the best of times. This is not an easy matter to face but one which cannot be ignored and it is worth saying at the outset that seeking early advice if you believe you are facing financial problems can save you worry later.

If you have a job and your ability to work is not too badly affected so that your employer continues to pay you as usual, a loss of income may not be an issue. If this is not the case, you will need to find out whether you are able to claim any State benefits to help you. You may find this difficult, particularly if you are accustomed to supporting your family financially, either alone or jointly. The idea that you are no longer able to guarantee to 'provide' for them in the same way is not easy to accept. In spite of this, it is important to ensure you receive any benefits you are entitled to – this is not a time to allow pride and your sense of independence from the State to stand in the way of financial help.

If you were not working or were retired, then your usual sources of income may be unaffected but it is nonetheless important for you to establish whether you are now entitled to any benefits as a result of your cancer.

You may feel disinclined to wade through booklets and forms when you already have enough on your mind. There is likely to be a social worker attached to your hospital whom you can consult for help in determining whether you qualify for any financial help. Do draw on their expertise – they may be able to save you time and effort by advising you and providing you with booklets and the relevant forms to fill in, and help you with the forms if you wish. If you prefer, information about Social Security is available by phone on Freeline Social Security 0800 666 555. The Benefit Enquiry Line on 0800 88 22 00 also exists for information on benefits for people who are sick or have a disability. The Benefits Agency produces a number of booklets containing information about these benefits, and you may be able to obtain these from your hospital.

For me initially the Benefits Agency appeared a complete mystery. I had never had any direct dealings with the DSS (from a personal rather than a business perspective) and their whole manner and method – not to mention the thickness and complexity of the application forms – was enough to make me feel that the whole exercise could not be worth the effort. The level of questioning and intrusion into what had previously been private matters was very disconcerting. However, I was very lucky to be referred to the hospital social worker who immediately – and correctly – identified those benefits to which I and my partner were entitled. (Neither of us was working now – I was not physically able to and my partner was spending all the time she could with me in hospital or supporting me at home.) The social worker also guided us through the application forms. The moral is to use the resources which are available to you as a patient. Do seek out the key social worker who will be on 'your side', don't accept any initial rejections by the Benefits Agency if you are sure you have a good case and hold out for those benefits to which you are legally and morally entitled.

The details which follow give an outline of the more common benefits available. They are not exhaustive, and you may be entitled to more help depending on your circumstances.

Statutory Sick Pay

If you are working, you will need to talk to your employer about your cancer and treatment, and whether you are likely to need time off work. It may be that your employer continues to pay you your normal salary. If not, you may be entitled to Statutory Sick Pay if you earn at least the lower earnings limit for Class 1 National Insurance contributions.

If you are not entitled to Statutory Sick Pay, then you may be able to claim Incapacity Benefit instead.

Incapacity Benefit

This is for people under State pension age whose employers do not pay Statutory Sick Pay, or who are self-employed, unemployed or non-employed. To qualify, you must satisfy certain criteria regarding your National Insurance contributions. There are various rates at which the benefit is paid:

- short-term Incapacity Benefit at the lower rate for up to 28 weeks;
- short-term Incapacity Benefit at the higher rate from weeks 29 to 52;
- long-term Incapacity Benefit after the end of 52 weeks (this is the highest rate).

If you are not expected to recover from your cancer then after 28 weeks you may qualify for the long-term rate. Depending on how serious your cancer is, you may find you are advised to apply for this level of benefit by virtue of the very nature of your treatment and the uncertainty which often surrounds the prognosis for someone being treated for cancer. It can still come as a shock to be classified as 'terminally ill' for the purpose of State benefits – do not feel you are being written off.

Any savings you or your wife or partner have do not affect your entitlement to Incapacity Benefit. However, this benefit does count towards your 'taxable income'.

If you do not qualify for Incapacity Benefit because you have not paid enough National Insurance contributions, you may be entitled to Severe Disablement Allowance.

Severe Disablement Allowance

This is for people who have been unable to work for at least 28 weeks and who have not paid enough National Insurance contributions to qualify for Incapacity Benefit. It is tax-free.

Disability Living Allowance

You may feel that this could not apply to you because you do not regard cancer as a 'disability'. For the purpose of this benefit, however, 'disability' is defined as requiring help with personal care or with mobility, or both. Disability Living Allowance is tax-free and is not affected by either your National Insurance contributions or your savings. It is generally for people under 65.

There are two quite distinct elements to the benefit. You may qualify for the 'personal care' element if you need help with, for example, washing, dressing and using the toilet, or preparing a cooked meal. The 'mobility' element may apply if you are unable or find it difficult to walk, or if you need someone with you when you walk to ensure your safety.

Under normal circumstances, you would not qualify for Disability Living Allowance until you have needed help for at least three months. There are however special rules for people with a terminal illness who may not live for longer than six months and you may qualify for your benefit immediately. It is of course accepted that even when people are not expected to recover, they may well live longer than six months. This does not affect your benefit – and does not mean that it will be withdrawn after six months.

The two elements of the benefit are considered separately, and are paid at different rates. There are three rates for the care element, and two for the mobility element. It is not necessary to claim for both elements in order to qualify – you can claim one or the other.

Attendance Allowance

This is for people aged 65 or over who need help with their personal care as a result of their illness. It is tax-free and it is not affected by either your National Insurance contributions or savings.

Usually, you would not qualify for this benefit until you have needed help for at least six months. However, special rules (as described above) apply for people with a terminal illness who may not live for longer than six months and under these rules you would receive your benefit more quickly.

There are two rates for this benefit:

- the lower rate for people who need help during the day *or* the night;
- the higher rate for people who need help during the day *and* the night.

Invalid Care Allowance

This is a benefit paid to a person who gives you a substantial amount of regular care. It is not affected by that person's National Insurance contributions, but that person must be of working age. To qualify, certain criteria must be met. You (the person being cared for) must be receiving:

- Disability Living Allowance care element at the middle or higher rate; or
- Constant Attendance Allowance at at least the normal maximum rate; or
- Attendance Allowance at either rate.

Additionally, the person caring for you must be:

- aged 16 to 65 when they claim;
- spending at least 35 hours a week caring for you;
- earning no more than £50 per week (after deducting allowable expenses);
- not attending full-time education (more than 21 hours per week).

The person caring for you may be able to claim more money if they are looking after your children or additional money for your children.

Depending on your circumstances, you might be entitled to other benefits such as:

- Income Support
- Family Credit
- Housing Benefit
- Council Tax Benefit

as well as help with the cost of prescriptions, hospital travel and other health-related expenses.

Again, you can either check for yourself in the Benefits Agency booklets, or ask to speak to the social worker at your hospital if you think you might qualify – or if you would just like to check exactly what you are entitled to claim.

Don't worry in silence

Money worries affect many people from time to time and your ability to cope with your cancer will not be helped if you are suffering the additional stress of wondering how you will pay your bills. This can place relationships under further strain at a time when solidarity is so important, and probably the worst course of action is to avoid the issue altogether. Both you and your wife or partner and family may be fully aware of potential problems without wanting to voice your fears and fuel an already stressful situation.

The only constructive solution is to talk to those who can help – particularly the social workers at your hospital (if there are none at your hospital, ask your GP for a referral). If you are already experiencing problems paying your bills, do contact the organizations in question and explain your circumstances. It will often be possible to negotiate a solution or compromise, but you will have to take the first step. It may be tempting to ignore your financial commitments in the hope that they will somehow disappear – but this is rarely the case. It may feel particularly harsh, but with some help and your own resolve, reasonable solutions can often be found.

Keeping your affairs in order

However good your prognosis, your cancer still represents – at best – a major scare in your life. However matter-of-fact and sensible we are, none of us cares to acknowledge our own mortality, but some circumstances do push us into considering whether our practical and financial affairs are in reasonable order.

Making a will

If you have not already made a will, then even if your prognosis is good, you may feel that this is a task you should put off no longer. You may still find the resolution to do so easier than actually tackling the task – but it *is* a very worthwhile exercise. It is often mistakenly believed that if your affairs are relatively simple then your assets will automatically pass to your wife or partner or children. This is not necessarily the case, and it is *much* better if you set down your wishes in writing. Not only does it make the task of administering your estate much more straightforward for your executors but it also gives you the opportunity to express any wishes you may have about bequests. A will does not have to be a complicated document. You can ask a solicitor to help you draw it up, or you may prefer to do it yourself from a ready-made 'kit' which you can obtain from stationers, or to use a book on the subject to devise your own will from scratch. *The Which? Guide to Wills and Probate* edited by the Consumers' Association is very useful. *The New Natural Death Handbook* also contains a good section of general guidance on wills. It may still be a good idea to ask a solicitor to check your will to ensure it is valid, unambiguous and would be legally acceptable.

Once your will is drawn up, you can forget about it (unless anything occurs in your life which necessitates changes). It is an important task dealt with.

> We had made our wills in an unusual burst of good sense while in our mid-20s, largely because I was in the process of setting up my business and we were not then married. They were very simple, and we typed them ourselves using a library book on wills and probate. When we received the news that my prognosis was looking much worse, we had another burst of sorting out our affairs and my partner (we were married five days later) made a panicky phone call to our local solicitor who kindly looked over our wills the same day and checked that they were 'legal' and contained no ambiguities. We hadn't realized that although they were basically fine as they stood, they would have become invalid after our marriage and were redrafted to take account of this. This was another item crossed off the list. We did not enjoy the process because of the implications, but it somehow felt like a small matter over which we still had some control and which we could sort out ourselves, and that is very important when it seems that everything else is running away from you.

You might also be spurred on to check that your financial and legal documents are accessible and reasonably well-organized. Again this is not an easy task to contemplate, and you may feel it is simply too much for you, or that somehow it is 'tempting fate'. If you can't manage it, fine – some people can and others can't. At first it may seem too overwhelming a task or you may feel that you need time to build up to it, but ensuring that your affairs are in good order can both relieve a potential source of worry and contribute to a sense of control on your part.

9
The aftermath – and the future

Reaching the end of your cancer treatment can bring tremendous relief – but also new and different uncertainties. For the duration of your treatment you have the framework in your life of hospital visits, check-ups and progress consultations. While this can be far from pleasant, it can provide a kind of reassurance, a sense that you are being constantly looked after and that your cancer is being attacked. The check-ups will continue, of course, but some men do find it difficult to adjust back to a life in which the focus of treatment is no longer present. This may be mixed with a huge sense of relief that you have arrived at the end of this stage and that you *have* coped with this experience.

If you were able to continue a relatively 'normal' life during your treatment, then you may feel less impact when it is completed. If you had to stop working or give up your normal routines, and found that your life was largely dominated by your cancer, then you will be facing a further period of transition. Going back to work or looking for a new job or picking up the threads of your life before cancer may feel like a huge task. You may in any case be limited by the advice of your medical team to take life gently for a while.

Some men find that living with cancer has given them a new or different outlook on life. Perhaps your sense of priorities has changed, or issues which previously seemed very important have become less so. Perhaps there have been subtle changes in relationships which cause you to value friends and loved ones more consciously. This does not imply that you have changed for the better as an individual – or changed at all.

You might see the end of your treatment as an opportunity to explore new directions in your life or to change the emphasis. Perhaps you feel that your career has a different significance now and that you want to spend more time pursuing other activities. This does not mean that you will always feel this way, but rather that your cancer has prompted you to reassess certain aspects of your life. If you do feel strongly that your priorities have changed dramatically and that you intend to make significant changes to your life then take the time to think these through, discuss them with your family and friends, and work out how you plan to use your time and energies. It is not uncommon to experience doubts and fears about how well you will cope. Will you manage to fulfil your role as husband/partner/father/son/friend as you did before your cancer? Will people regard you differently now? There will obviously be continuing concern for your well-being, and you may feel frustrated that people still dwell on your cancer for some time.

You may also experience fears about the recurrence of your cancer. This is an issue which will not go away, and while doctors would dearly like to give you watertight guarantees for the future, this is just not possible. You may feel that you simply want to put the whole experience behind you, forget about it and get back to 'real' life again. You would not be human if you did not have fears and doubts, though. You *are* allowed to be worried and anxious, but it is important not to bottle up your fears unnecessarily. Talk to those close to you – they are almost certainly sharing exactly the same anxieties, and will welcome the chance to say so and to let you know that they are willing you on to a full recovery. If you find that you are becoming over-anxious or depressed about the future, then do not hesitate to contact your GP or ask at your hospital about counselling. Specialist cancer counsellors often provide continuing support – after all, the end of your treatment does not mean that your experience of cancer simply comes to an abrupt end. If you need to talk further, then allow yourself to do so.

Gary was surprised by feelings of guilt after radiotherapy treatment for his brain tumour proved more successful than was originally anticipated. He felt guilty that the treatment had worked for him, but that others around him were less fortunate, and began thinking, 'How is it that I have survived when others are dying?' He had undergone regular counselling throughout his treatment, and found it useful to discuss his feelings with his counsellor.

You may experience an unexpected sense of frustration, as Neil found:

I began to feel intensely frustrated soon after the final chemotherapy session of my initial treatment. It was late in the year, and I decided to give myself to the end of that year to recuperate and decide 'what to do next'. I had previously been running my own business, practising as a chartered accountant, but sold the practice soon after my diagnosis. The first few days of the following January were not easy because there was no obvious new path to take, yet I was feeling strong and well and wanted to start working on something positive and constructive immediately. I knew, of course, that it can take time for new projects to emerge – which, in fact, they quickly did – and in the intervening period, I felt as if I was treading water when I wanted to be swimming the Channel. All I can say is try to hang on and be patient (I wasn't, particularly!) – it *is* frustrating.

Life does go on after cancer. It may have caused big changes in your life or it may have had less impact. There is no right way to view your experience – some men choose to try to find some constructive element on which they can draw in the future and others want to try to forget about it as soon as possible. Returning to 'normal' may be a long process, and 'normal' may mean something different to you now.

Any journey through cancer treatment is hard, and inevitably it will leave its mark. But it is possible to make a positive difference by resolving to manage with determination and, together with family and friends, to confront and take what control you can of such an unwelcome situation. Above all, be aware of your achievement in coping with your cancer and congratulate yourself on reaching each milestone in your treatment.

Glossary of medical terms

It will help if you become familiar with certain medical terms, because you will hear them used by your medical team and an understanding of their meaning will help you to feel more involved in your treatment and in control of conversations and consultations.

The following list is not intended to be exhaustive, but includes the commoner terms and jargon you may encounter. If you are in doubt about the terms your medical team use, never be afraid to ask them for explanations.

Adenocarcinoma
A relatively common form of cancer which starts in a gland, e.g. breast or bowel.

Adjuvant therapy
After surgery to remove a tumour, there may be no trace of cancer remaining. Adjuvant therapy such as radiotherapy or chemotherapy may be given to reduce the chance of the cancer returning.

Analgesic
Pain-killing drug.

Ascites
A build-up of fluid in the abdomen, causing swelling and often discomfort and/or breathlessness.

Barium enema
A type of X-ray in which a barium liquid is introduced into the rectum before an X-ray is taken in which the barium shows up white.

Biopsy
A specimen of tissue taken for examination under a microscope to check for the presence of abnormal cells, which will facilitate diagnosis.

Carcinogen
A substance capable of causing cancer.

Carcinoma
A cancer which originates in the epithelial tissue. The most common type of cancer.

CT or CAT scan
Stands for Computerized Tomography or Computerized Axial Tomography. A form of X-ray which gives clearer and more detailed images than conventional X-ray.

Cytotoxic
'Cell-poisoning' drugs used in chemotherapy for the treatment of cancer.

Endoscopy
A procedure in which a thin tube is used to look inside a part of the body – the stomach, bladder, bowel, lungs, for example.

Epithelium
The layer of cells which covers (such as the skin) or provides the lining of organs (such as the stomach or bowel).

Hormone
A substance produced by one of the body's glands, which is released into the bloodstream and affects the function of another organ.

IVP
Stands for Intravenous Pyelogram, an X-ray of the kidneys and urinary system using a dye to highlight the organs.

Localized tumour
A cancer which has not spread beyond the site in which it originated.

Lymphogram
An X-ray which uses dye to show up the lymph nodes as it flows through the lymph channels, used to detect enlarged lymph nodes.

Mediastinoscopy
An examination in which a thin tube is used to look at and take biopsies of the tissue in the centre of the chest between the lungs.

Metastasis
The process whereby a cancer spreads and invades tissues in distant parts of the body from the primary tumour, often via the bloodstream or lymphatic system. It forms secondary tumours, which generally behave like the primary tumour and which therefore respond to the same treatment.

MRI scan
Stands for Magnetic Resonance Imaging. A means of using magnetic fields rather than X-rays to produce very clear images of the body.

Neo-adjuvant therapy
This refers to therapy given before surgery with the intention of reducing the tumour size and making surgery easier to perform.

Neoplasm
Also referred to as a tumour, a lump or growth of cells.

Oncogene
A gene which has the properties to cause a cell to become malignant. Most are mutant forms of genes which are essential for normal cellular growth and development.

Oncologist
A doctor who specializes in cancer.

Palliative treatment
Treatment whose aim is to alleviate the symptoms of cancer but not to cure the cancer.

Platelets
One of the constituents of blood which affects the blood's clotting ability.

Radiographer
A specialist who operates the machines which administer radio-therapy treatment.

Radiologist
A specialist dealing with X-rays.

Recurrence/relapse
The return of a detectable cancer after treatment and a period of remission.

Remission
The lack of any detectable cancer and disappearance of symptoms.

Sarcoma
A cancer which originates in the bone, muscle or other connective tissues such as tendon and cartilage.

Systemic
Involving the whole body, not just a localized area.

Tumour
A lump or growth caused by a mass of cells. Can be benign if it is non-invasive or malignant if invasive. See also neoplasm.

Tumour markers
Substances which are produced by certain cancers and are detectable in the bloodstream. They are used for the purposes of diagnosis and monitoring the progress of treatment.

Ultrasound
A completely harmless means of using high frequency sound waves to produce an image of the inside of the body. (As used on pregnant women to visualize their baby.)

Useful contacts

BACUP (British Association of Cancer United Patients)
3 Bath Place
Rivington Street
London
EC2A 3JR
Tel: 0171 696 9003
Publishes booklets on different types of cancer and aspects of living with cancer.

BACUP Cancer Information Service
Tel: 0171 613 2121
Freephone (outside London): 0800 181 199
Mon–Thurs 10am–7pm, Fri 10am–5.30pm
Specially trained cancer nurses answer queries by phone about all aspects of living with cancer.

BACUP Cancer Counselling Service
London-based, *tel*: 0171 696 9000, or Glasgow-based, *tel*: 0141 553 1553
Professional counsellors available to talk through the problems which can arise from living with cancer. Free and confidential, phone for an appointment.

CancerLink
17 Britannia Street   9 Castle Street
London   Edinburgh
WC1X 9JN   EH1 2DP
Tel: 0171 833 2451   *Tel*: 0131 228 5557
Mon–Fri 9.30am–5pm
Information and support, by phone or letter, on all aspects of cancer. Publishes an annual *Directory of Cancer Support and Self Help*, and a range of publications on cancer.

131

Cancer Relief Macmillan Fund
16–19 Britten Street
London
SW3 3TZ
Tel: 0171 351 7811
Provides financial grants in certain circumstances for people living with cancer and their families. Home care nurses available through the Macmillan service.

Marie Curie Cancer Care
28 Belgrave Square
London
SW1X 8QG
Tel: 0171 235 3325
Home nursing service for people with cancer, free of charge. Care centres throughout the UK.

The Help for Health Trust
Freephone: 0800 66 55 44
Mon–Fri 9am–5pm
Free, confidential health information (not specific medical advice), including details of self-help and support groups and a leaflet library.

Hospice Information Service
St Christopher's Hospice
Lawrie Park Road
Sydenham
London
SE26 6DZ
Tel: 0181 778 9252
Produces a *Directory of Hospice Services* – in-patient, home care and hospital support teams in the UK and Eire.

The Natural Death Centre
20 Heber Road
London
NW2 6AA
Tel: 0181 208 2853
An educational charity which publishes *The New Natural Death Handbook* and works to support those dying at home.

Websites
BACUP
http://www.cancerbacup.org.uk
Information about cancer and treatments, support groups and cancer organizations.

Imperial Cancer Research Fund
http://www.icnet.uk
Information about cancer research and fundraising.

National Cancer Institute (USA)
http://www.gustav@imsdd.meb.uni-bonn.de
http://www.pueschel@imsdd.meb.uni-bonn.de
http://www.far@imsdd.meb.uni-bonn.de
CancerNet 'PDQ' database with up-to-date information about cancer prevention, detection, treatment and care.

Index